Natural Health Care for Your Dog

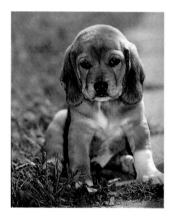

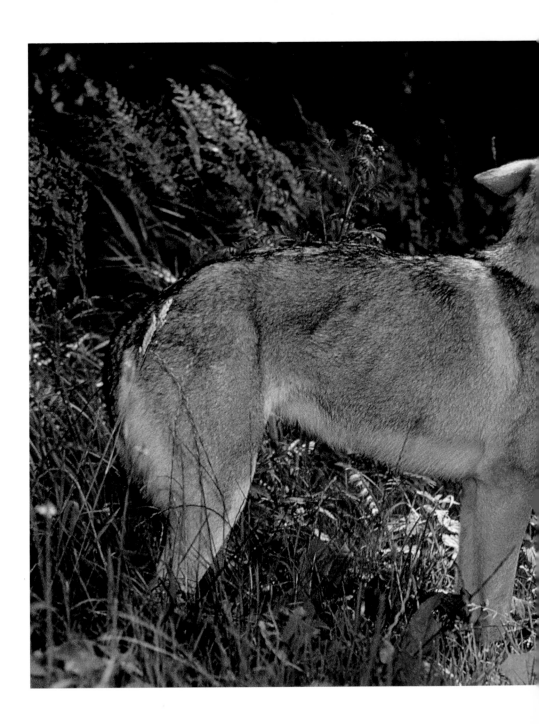

Petra Stein

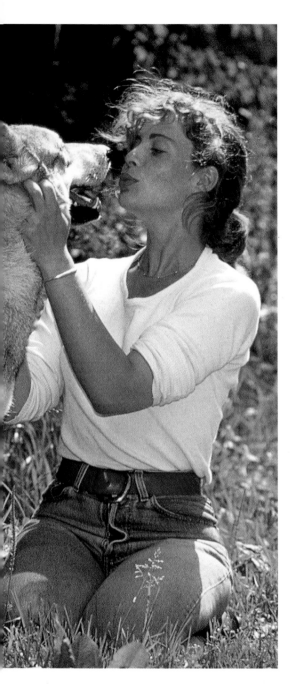

Natural Health Care for Your
Dog

Quick Self-Help Using
Homeopathy and Bach Flowers

Color Photography by Monika Wegler

Drawings by György Jankovics

BARRON'S

Contents

Treating Diseases at Home
Pages 32–97 (see page 5)

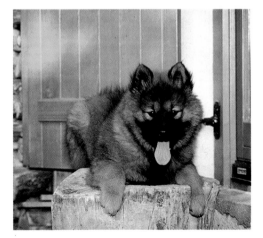

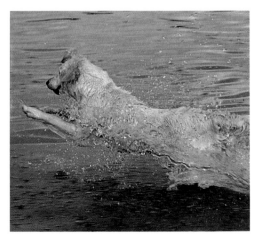

Practical Advice for Dog Owners

Appendix

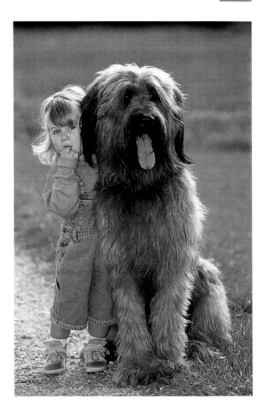

Treating Diseases at Home

What You Should Know About Your Dog

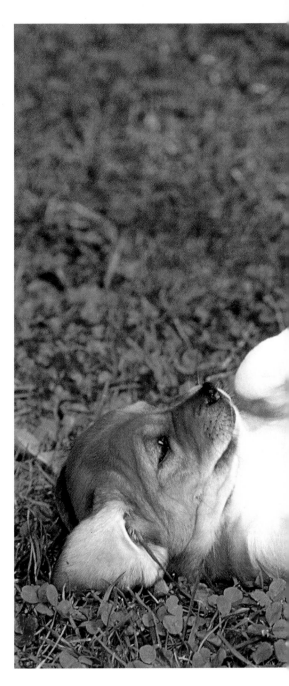

Growing up with dogs is an experience you don't want to miss as it prepares you for a life with dogs as companions. Dogs become partners in life and in play, they serve as watchdogs, they accompany you on walks, and later in life, they become welcome listeners when you are alone.

Of course, as a pet owner, you must take responsibility for your dog. This does not consist of merely feeding your pet and providing it a place to sleep. Your responsibility includes spending quality time with your dog and caring for the animal in all the ways necessary to keep the animal well.

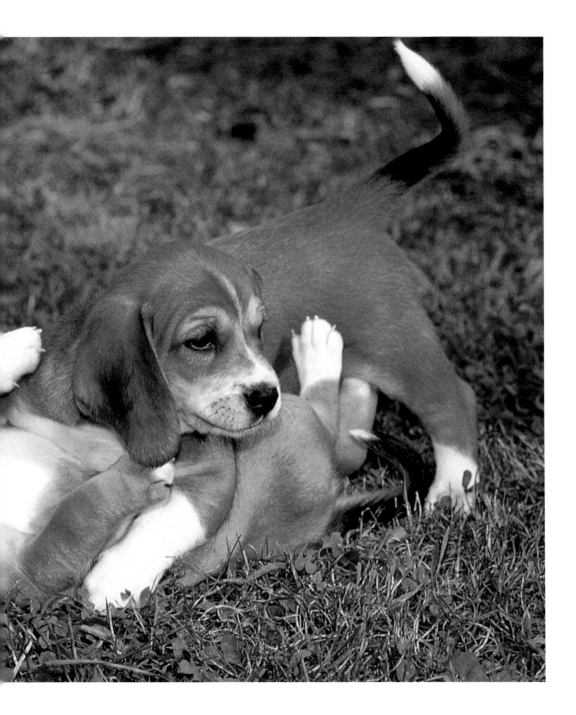

Preventive Health Care

Scheduling Preventive Care

Most of us humans are used to going to a doctor for an annual checkup. This is a useful thing to do because it helps us to recognize potential health problems before they turn into full-blown diseases, and it spares the body the extra work of having to cope with a multitude of sick organ systems. The same idea should be applied to your four-legged friends. Every good veterinarian will perform a general exam and a quick fecal test, even when you visit the clinic "only" for vaccination boosters. You should, also, present your dog annually to a natural health care specialist who is able to perform a *bio-resonance analysis* (see pages 24–25). This test will indicate predispositions or increased susceptibilities to potential diseases. We all know that the earlier we recognize any illness, the higher the chances are for effective treatments. The same is true for your dog.

Tick Prevention

Ticks are most actively prevalent during the spring and autumn. Female ticks transmit serious diseases because they suck blood from their bite victim (see page 79). If you give your dog Preparation-Z Tablets, you can protect your dog from this risk. The pills contain minerals, vitamins, and dried meat products, which, when combined, produce a type of skin exudate that repels ticks. It is not a smell that is perceptible to humans. The usual commercial tick collars contain chemicals that are absorbed through the skin. These chemicals reach the general metabolic pathways and can cause problems along their way through the body.

Worm Prevention

A common source of worm infestation is raw meat that was neither fresh-frozen nor released for human consumption (see page 56).

You should have your dog's stool examined *twice yearly* for worm infestation. When you take your dog to a veterinarian trained in holistic techniques for a checkup, a stool examination is routinely part of the procedure. If the result is negative, you only need to treat your dog for ten days with five to ten drops of Tanacet-Heel daily. This treatment will discourage internal parasites from settling in the dog's intestines.

A full-fledged worming treatment is necessary only if the stool exam is positive for worms. In this case, the veterinarian will prescribe a product that will eliminate endoparasites without harming the intestines or their natural bacterial flora.

Vaccination Schedule

✓ **2–6 weeks:** *(Orphan puppies that did not receive colostrum)* Distemper-Hepatitis, Parvovirus, Leptospirosis, Parainfluenza
✓ **8 weeks:** Distemper-Hepatitis, Parvovirus, Leptospirosis, Parainfluenza
✓ **12 weeks:** Distemper-Hepatitis, Parvovirus, Leptospirosis, Parainfluenza
✓ **3–4 months:** Rabies, Distemper-Hepatitis, Parvovirus, Leptospirosis, Parainfluenza
✓ **Beginning at 1 year** [Every 3rd year (or as required by local laws)]: Rabies
✓ **Yearly:** Distemper-Hepatitis, Parvovirus, Leptospirosis, Parainfluenza

Dogs sniff the ground to gather information, but in doing so they also pick up many disease-causing agents.

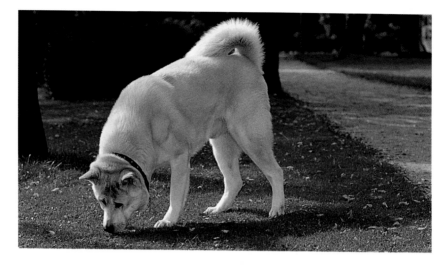

Regular Vaccination Schedules

Infectious diseases are best prevented by getting your dog vaccinated on a regular booster schedule. This is done by veterinarians.

Puppies are protected by maternal antibodies until they are eight weeks old. At this time you should begin the immunization schedule as outlined on page 8.

Remember that you will need a rabies vaccination certificate when you cross the border into a foreign country.

Kennel cough is a disease that mainly affects dogs that are frequently housed in group kennels. If your dog lives exclusively in your home, you can skip this immunization.

What Causes Diseases?

There are many internal and external causes of disease, and psychological problems are among them.

Among the *external causes of disease* are bacteria, viruses, fungi, moisture, cold temperatures, and a host of ever-increasing environmental stimuli, such as noise and smog. *Internal causes of*

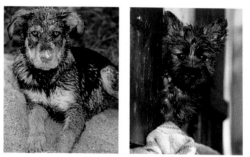

Playfulness and curiosity are the hallmarks of healthy dogs.

disease are just as numerous. They include improper diet, ingestion of toxic substances, and complex factors that are caused by poor genetic control during the breed selection processes. Genetic causes are observed in some purebred dogs more than in others. Dogs of these breeds are predisposed to certain illnesses from the day they are born.

Psychological disturbances not only increase a dog's susceptibility to disease but also lower the ability to fight illness by natural healing processes.

Positive Interaction

It should be understood by every pet owner that all aspects of care and handling must be optimal to yield a healthy and happy dog.

The Well-Balanced Human–Animal Bond

Before you acquire a dog, you should consider carefully whether you will be able to spend sufficient time with your pet. If you are frequently away from your home and if you know that you are unable to take a dog along with you, then you should decide against this type of pet ownership. This decision will spare you and the dog much distress. Dogs have evolved as pack animals. They suffer when they are left alone for extended periods.

Train your dog gently and with consistency. The earlier your pet understands you and you understand your pet, the simpler and closer your future will be together. Puppies learn just about everything easily when they are trained in a playful manner; and a well-trained pet is sure to form a harmonious bond with its master. While your dog is young, instructions are absorbed without an urge to resist or counteract commands.

Always remember the reward for each successful task your pet has completed!

Never punish your dog when it seeks your presence after having committed a misdeed. Dogs are unable to connect their actions with your punishment, and your pet will relate your anger solely to your personality, leaving the animal confused and distraught. Once a dog loses trust in its owner, the loss is hard to repair. You may punish your dog only when you are present at the moment your dog commits a misdeed. Never hit your dog with your hands because your hands should be trusted as providing praise, pets, and cuddles.

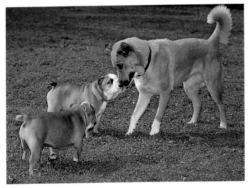

The nose serves as a first contact point between unfamiliar dogs.

Proper Husbandry and Care

Once daily
- ✓ Brushing
- ✓ Eye care
- ✓ Teeth cleaning

After every walk
- ✓ Cleaning of the nose pad
- ✓ Taking care of the paws
- ✓ Checking anal and genital areas

Weekly
- ✓ Ear care

When needed
- ✓ Nail care
- ✓ Bathing

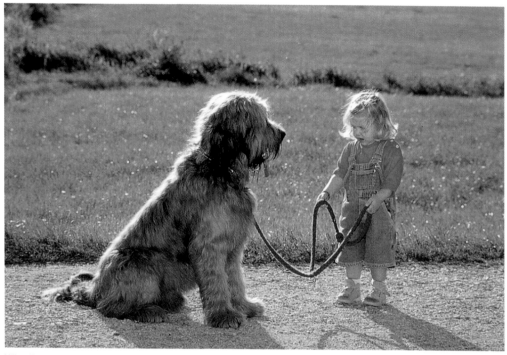

Who do you think will get his way here?

Play with your dog as much as you possibly can and talk to the animal like you do to a friend. Your dog will soon respond in its own particular body language.

When you decide to get a second dog, you must make sure that you pay equal attention to both spend equal time with them and make sure that one does not get preferential treatment over the other. If you are not careful, you will produce feelings of jealousy or anger, and harmony will be difficult to maintain in the long run.

The Bond Between Child and Dog

If you had a chance to grow up with pets, you understand the value and joy of friendships between children and dogs. This is a great way for children to learn how to take care of an animal responsibly.

No matter how positive your child's interaction with the dog might be, you must pay attention to these reminders:

● You will be guilty of *negligence* if you leave your child alone with a dog, no matter how small or gentle your dog! Any animal may behave unpredictably in unanticipated situations!

● Prevent the risk of parasite transmission from dog to child by regular fecal examinations.

Providing the Right Care for Your Dog

As you know, wolves are our dog's ancestors. From these origins our domestic dogs have retained several behavioral traits. They have remained pack animals who need to feel that they are part of a fixed hierarchical order and who will accept any customs submissively if they are taught their place in the pack. For you, the dog owner, this means that you should try to provide a certain degree of routine daily patterns while being sensitive to the particular needs of your canine friend.

A Place for Your Dog

A place just for your dog is very important for its well-being. Dogs need a place to which they can retreat when they need to be alone. The best of all choices would be a spot that was chosen by the animal itself, but in many modern small apartments this option is just not available. Remember, however, that if you observe that your dog just does not seem to accept the place you choose, this does not mean that your dog is a bad dog who does not follow orders. Your dog is probably instinctively refusing a drafty location or one with too much walking traffic or an exposure to electromagnetic fields. Accept your pet's sensitivities, and find a more suitable place for its resting needs.

The chosen spot should be prepared according to its size and in the form of a basket or a large enough foam mattress pad. Cover the lair with a blanket or towels. These covers should be washed weekly to prevent bacterial contamination.

Kenneling dogs outside should only be a choice for very specific watchdog requirements. Chaining dogs is nothing short of a crime. It is no wonder that these dogs are bound to become aggressive.

A Place for Food and Water

From the beginning, let your dog know that food and water bowls are always in the same place. The feeding area should be easily sanitizable because dogs spill food when they eat. Meticulous cleanliness of the food bowls is essential to maintain the health of your dog.

A dog should be allowed to eat its food undisturbed. For feeding times and food amounts, see page 16.

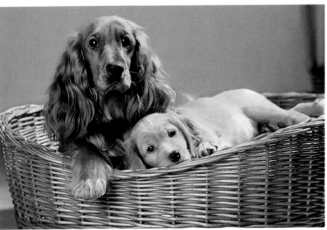

Cuddles in Mom's basket is true happiness for this puppy.

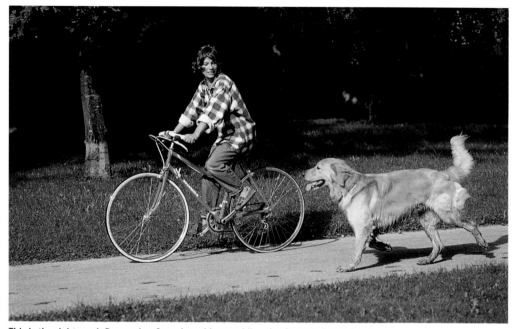

This is the right way! By running free alongside your bike, the dog can determine its own speed.

The Daily Walk

From their wolf forefathers dogs have retained the need for lots of running activities. This need must be satisfied daily in order to assure your dog a long and healthy life with you.

Three to four daily outings should be the basic plan of activity for your dog. This activity is also needed for regular bowel movements and for urine elimination. Walks and outings can be long or short depending on the size and breed of your dog. The closer you observe your animal, the better you can judge the particular needs of your four-legged friend.

While your dog is still a puppy, it is best to take it outside shortly after each meal. This way the puppy will eliminate before it will curl up for a restful snooze.

For your adult dog, it will be more interesting if you vary the walking routes. Take different roads for long and short walks.

As long as you provide sufficient outdoor activity, you can be sure that even a large dog is happy and healthy in a small apartment. This means, however, that you will need to plan three hours of walks or outdoor activity every day.

Good Nutrition

"The way to a person's heart is through his/her stomach." This saying is as true for dogs as it is for humans. A menu that lists the same meal for every day can bore even the most patient dog.

Make your dog's meal a happy, creative, and interesting affair by offering a variety of nutritionally rich and balanced meals. The world of advertisements can spin your head with names and promises while you must ask one simple question, "What is the right food for my dog?"

Which Food?

There is no patented answer to this question. First you must decide whether you want to cook meals for your dog or you prefer commercial diets. If your time is limited, the latter will be your only choice.

When you choose a commercial canned food, you should pay attention to the meat listed in the ingredients. Dogs are not vegetarians and the meat component must be high enough. Also, choose a food that is low or devoid of chemical additives. This includes chemicals added for preservation, color, or taste enhancements. Many dogs are allergic to a variety of these ingredients and long term feeding of certain food additives can lead to severe metabolic complications.

If you have dogs and cats in your home, you should take special care to feed them separately. Because of the different protein requirements, it is frequently observed that dogs have allergic reactions to cat foods.

If you choose to exclusively feed dry kibbled food, you must check regularly that your dog is provided with, and drinks, ample amounts of water to prevent kidney problems. With dry food

Home Cooked Meals

Raw meats
✓ beef: tripe, heart, other parts
✓ veal, lamb

Cooked meats
✓ poultry (carefully boned)
✓ game, venison

Cooked fish
✓ seabass, halibut, shellfish (remove all bones carefully)

Cooked, chopped vegetables
✓ fennel, chicory, spinach, carrots, zucchini

Herbs
✓ parsley, caraway, sage, chives, some garlic

and canned food, it is important that you pay close attention to the type and amount of any chemical additives.

How to Prepare Well-Balanced Home Cooked Meals for Your Dog

If you love to cook and you have sufficient time, your dog will love you for your home cooked meals. *Raw meats* are the most nutritional foods for dogs. You must assure yourself of the quality and freshness of the meats and you must make sure that the meat is fresh-frozen for human consumption. This added attention will pay off by keeping your dog free of worms.

The food guide that follows lists foods that you can choose for your dog. There are a variety of

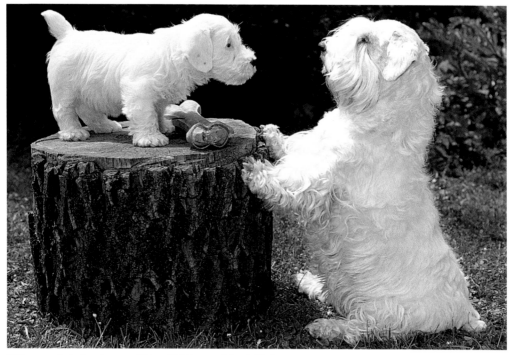

Still young, but already sure of himself, this pup defends his bone.

food items that you can add to the regular meals: You can use unprocessed rice, which requires extended cooking time, or you can use oatmeal, pasta, cottage cheese, or low fat cottage cheese. If the nutritional composition is not well balanced, you can be sure that metabolic problems will occur, which will lead to skin and coat changes or to digestive tract illnesses.

Important: Do *not* feed pork meats at any time. Aujeszkey disease is fatal and pork meats have been implicated as the cause of the problem.

Avoid	Because
Too many bones	Constipation, intestinal blockage (potentially fatal)
Bones of poultry and game	Danger of injuries to the esophagus and intestines
Food leftovers and spiced foods	Kidney damage
Milk	Diarrhea
Beans	Gas; difficult to digest; low nutritional value
Sweets	Digestive problems
Snacks	Train dogs to beg

Food: How Much and When?

Consistent feeding routines are essential. Your dog should learn that you will provide food everyday at the same time and in the same location. This pattern will teach your pet to trust you, and it will prevent a behavioral pattern that says "I am waiting for food."

The amount of food varies with the size and temperament of the dog. A calm, slowly moving animal will need less food than a lively, active, and sports oriented dog.

Offer your dog a bowl of food. If anything is left over, the amount was too large. Feed less next time. If, however, your friend inhales the food in no time, looking for more, you should evaluate the animals' overall condition and make a decision as to whether hunger or greed is at work. Examine your dog carefully by feeling all parts of its body. You should "feel" the ribs but you should not be able to "count" them. The latter tells you to increase the food ration for your friend.

Whenever you find any inadvertent food leftovers, discard them. Leftovers may invite bacterial growth and should be avoided. Spoiled foods can lead to intestinal problems.

Feeding a Young Dog

A puppy is usually twelve weeks old when you take it home. If you have decided to provide home cooked meals, you need to find out exactly what type of food the puppy is used to. Changes in the food types, like changing from commercial to fresh meals, must be undertaken *slowly*, little by little. The intestinal tract of a puppy is not fully developed and it will react with diarrhea to any sudden food changes.

The basic components of puppy food are the same as those for adult dogs. The only differences are the proportions and the meal size (see table below). In addition, a puppy should receive a daily small amount of bone meal and Welpisal (dosage according to size).

These supplements strengthen the growth phase of the little body. In order to aid the general condition of the growing puppy, you should add a homeopathic supplement in the form of a high potentiated homeopathic remedy.

According to the general type and body structure of your dog, choose Calcium phosphoricum if your dog is slender and fine-boned, and use Calcium carbonicum if your dog is robust,

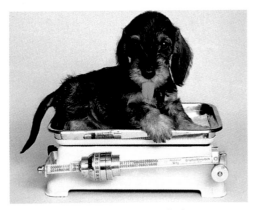

Feeding the right amount prevents obesity.

Feeding Schedule (daily requirements)

Age (in months)	Meals each day	Proportions of Meat to Other Ingredients
3rd–5th	4x	$^2/_3 : {}^1/_3$
5th–12th	3x	$^2/_3 : {}^1/_3$
from 12th	2x	$^1/_2 : {}^1/_2$
older dogs, sick dogs	3x	$^1/_3 : {}^2/_3$

strong, and muscular. In this case, you administer the product once only, because it is not a treatment for a disease condition. Since individual dogs vary so greatly in type and structure, ask your veterinarian trained in holistic techniques for the dosage that is correct for your particular puppy.

Nutrition for Sick Dogs

In order to assist the body's recovery process, it is important to feed sick dogs with a specific diet (see page 106).

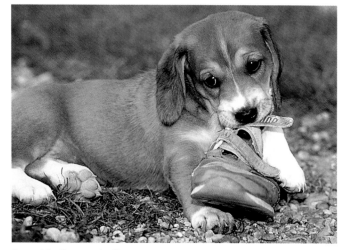

A great tasting sneaker?

Fluid Intake

For dogs it is more important to drink than to eat. Fluid intake keeps the kidneys functioning, which is essential for the body's detoxification. A dog can get along fine without food for a few days, but not without water! If you have a dog who drinks little by nature, make it a habit to add more moisture to its food. This will balance the need for fluids.

Always offer fresh clean water for drinking. Milk is not a substitute and it can cause diarrhea.

The amount of drinking water is determined individually by each dog. A small dog needs less than a large dog, and dogs who live on dry, kibbled food will need to drink more than those who get more canned, moist foods. You may try to get your dog used to a routine whereby you offer a large bowl of water after each walk and after each meal.

If the water is not fully consumed, discard the rest. You will soon learn how much your dog wants to drink.

Important: Pay special attention to renewing the drinking water regularly. If left in the bowl for more than one day, water will attract the growth of bacteria. This danger is increased during the warm summer months.

Home Remedies: An Overview

Natural or *holistic* medicine is the umbrella term to describe all treatments that use natural products and natural methods to preserve and stimulate health and healing through the body's own functions and defense mechanisms. Included are treatment procedures that unblock psychological or organic systems in order to reestablish their self-healing capacity. Also included are methods that work by aiding the regenerative powers of damaged organ and cell systems.

Natural health care for animals uses the knowledge and experience learned from human use of natural health remedies.

The education of a veterinarian trained in holistic techniques focuses on the primary diagnostic skills and on the ability of matching a natural medicinal preparation with the diagnosed disorder. Part of this specific training centers on the veterinarian's recognition of whether or not an animal is able or willing to respond to treatments by encouraging its own body's participation in the healing process. An animal's cooperation is essential in the success of the treatment. The educational program includes a wide variety of natural treatment methods, theories, and medicinal compounds. As practitioners, each specialist refines a certain type and number of methods in their treatment applications, rather than trying to practice all of the available treatment options.

We will now describe the treatments and products that are suggested for home use.

Homeopathy

Homeopathy is one of the essential components of this medical knowledge. The founder, Samuel Hahnemann (1755–1843) recognized the following: When a healthy body is exposed to a concentrated dose of certain substances, it will react with disease; however, if the same body is treated with a homeopathically potentiated form of the same substance, the disease is cured. The following is a typical example. Treat the symptoms of a bee sting with a homeopathic dose of Apis, which is extracted from bee sting poison (i.e., Apis), and you will see the symptoms recede.

The ingredients of the many treatments include minerals, plants, animal products, poisons, metals, and inorganic acids. *You can obtain all of these products in your pharmacy.* They are available in the form of tablets, powders, liquids, drops, globules, and ampules for oral administration.

Ampules are preferred because:
● They do not contain alcohol and they are of neutral taste, which is immensely important for sensitive animals and conditions that include inflammation inside the mouth. There is no pain and no burning sensation.
● They need to be taken only once daily.
● The Potentiation Accord, which has determined a set dilution factor for homeopathic single remedies, increases the overall effect on the body's own abilities. Medicines are formulated in homeopathic dilutions to effect specific results. Hahnemann had recognized that there was a proportional increase of healing with the degree of dilution of a medication. In order to express this seemingly opposite effect, Hahnemann used the term "potentiating" instead of "diluting."

As was mentioned above, a single-strength "potentiated" medication, if administered to a healthy body, will cause symptoms of disorder; but, administered to a diseased organism, the same single remedy will initiate a cure.

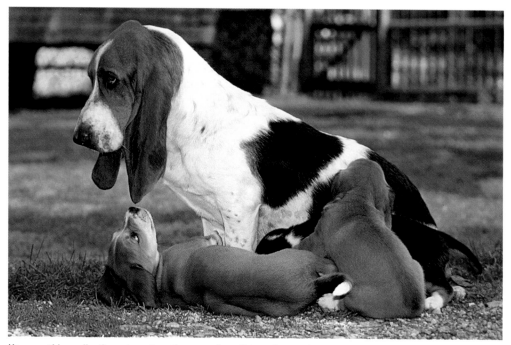

Homeopathic medications strengthen the general condition of a growing puppy.

The collective spectrum of symptoms that arises from the administration of a homeopathic substance is called the "medication syndrome." A veterinarian trained in holistic techniques must first find the right medication syndrome to arrive at a specific choice of medicinal substances that will match the characteristics of the targeted disease.

Bach Flower Therapy

Bach Flower therapy is designed to treat disharmonious conditions of the psyche and/or behavioral patterns in humans and animals.

Dr. Edward Bach founded this form of therapy about seventy years ago for human use. Today it is also used for the treatment of animals. According to Dr. Bach, a disease occurs in order to recreate harmony between body and soul. In animals, as in humans, there are many reasons to believe that a negative psychological environment can not only delay recovery from diseases, but can actually cause organic disease.

Bach Flower therapy recreates a positive balance for a negative body-mind condition of the animal. In dogs, it is difficult to recognize disease in its very early stages. Therefore, Bach Flowers are not considered to be curative medications in themselves, but are immensely important aids in the support of the organism, keeping it from further deterioration and from allowing disorders to extend into the realm of the psyche.

Bach Flowers constitute a complete health care system consisting of 38 different flowers and of one complex and concentrated mixture of many flowers, named "Rescue drops." Dr. Bach assigned each of the flower preparations for the treatment of 38 different conditions of the psyche. With the help of special extraction methods, the positive energies of the flowers are transferred to spring water. Subsequently, the water is preserved with alcohol or vinegar and stored in bottles. Bach Flowers are sold without restrictions through pharmacies. The drops are sold in 10 ml vials, except for the Rescue drops, which are sold in 20 ml vials.

The concentrated drops must be diluted with noncarbonated water before use. If several flower preparations are indicated for treatment at the same time, you need to mix them before use. Pharmacies frequently sell premixed Bach Flower combinations that are diluted in water as well as in alcohol.

Diluting the Concentrates:
(use bottled spring water)
To   Add
10 ml water : 2 drops of each flower
20 ml water : 4 drops of each flower
30 ml water : 6 drops of each flower
50 ml water : 8 drops of each flower

Preservatives are not needed up to a volume of 50 ml because the concentrated drops are based in alcohol. Mixtures may be used down to the last drop.

Exception:
Rescue drops should be used only in cases of emergency and for specific conditions. They are not intended for continued administration. A vial of 10 ml is usually sufficient for any treatment. Use five drops of concentrate in 10 ml bottled spring water.

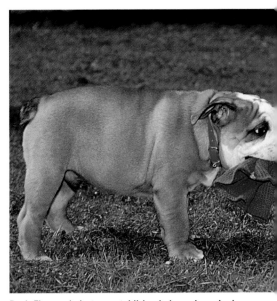

Bach Flowers help to reestablish a balanced psyche in a behaviorally disturbed dog.

Nosode Therapy

This therapy uses the body's own components, e.g., blood, urine, and secretions, to effect healing. Autologous blood treatments are included in this type of therapy. The basic theory of this method is to "treat like with like."

Nosode therapy represents the most intensive method of stimulating the body's own defensive mechanisms. Metabolic disorders are often covered up by other disturbances to the point where the original problem can no longer be recognized. Nosode therapy is used to change a chronic condition into an acute stage which can be treated by a variety of specific formulations.

It is important to understand that the use of Nosodes necessarily elicits a first phase during which all symptoms are aggravated. This problem

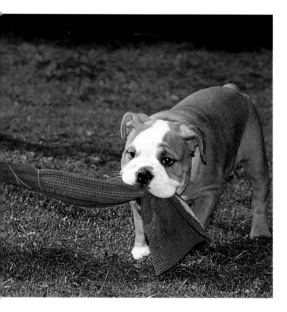

can be avoided by the administration of *Foreign Nosodes*, which are prepared from substrates of other animals rather than the body's own. These products are potentiated homeopathically and offered in the form of drops or ampules for oral administration. Potentiation helps to eliminate the stage of symptomatic aggravation. In the treatment of animals, this is particularly important because they cannot understand that their disease has to get just a little worse before it can get better. Another unique quality of the Foreign Nosode therapy is the effectiveness in eliminating toxins from the body using its own functions and, in so doing, unburdening the liver, kidney, intestines, and skin.

Cytoplasm Therapy
This method of healing enables the body to *regenerate* diseased areas of an organ system. The treatment elicits no side effects contrary to the commonly used "fresh-cell therapy," which has to

contend with allergic reactions, painful infections, fever, and apathy. In addition, this therapy does not require that the patient be quiet or restricted in any way, which is difficult to accomplish with a dog. Cytoplasm therapy is based on procedures that purify *fresh-cell* substrates by eliminating all components other than those that are effectively participating in regenerative processes.

Laser Acupuncture
Acupuncture is based on an old Chinese philosophy that a body incorporates two opposing forces, the yin and yang. Health was considered possible only if these forces were in balance. The flow of energy along specific lines (meridians) in our bodies may be interrupted by certain disorders that create blockages. The use of acupuncture can stimulate and free blockages along meridians. This rebalances the yin and yang. Originally, acupuncture was performed by the use of needles that were inserted along the meridians and remained in position for about 20 minutes. Today, this procedure is largely replaced by an infrared laser technique, which makes this a completely painless treatment. In addition, the use of lasers requires less time than the needles.

Acupressure
Acupressure is similar to the acupuncture method in that finger pressure is exerted on certain points of the body, thus stimulating a specific site. These sites are in the identical locations as those of acupuncture. Finger pressure elicits a similar, but less pronounced, reaction to that of needles or lasers.

This is a very useful technique that can be used at home to complement acupuncture treatment. The practitioner will instruct the dog owner in the use of this procedure.

Color Therapy
A variety of organic disorders can be affected positively by the exposure to colored lights. As

a rule, this method utilizes forty-watt colored lightbulbs that are placed at a certain distance from the animal. This technique does not depend on heat, but on the actual color light waves emitted, which have the ability to stimulate the body's own healing powers (see page 120).

Color therapy can be used at home as a complementary healing aid to other treatments. Your holistic specialist will instruct you in the specific choice of color spectrum you need to apply. Generally, greens and blues are used to treat hyperactive functions of the body, while organ functions that are too low are treated with yellow or red color ranges. For disorders of the nervous system, purple lights are used. There are also conditions where several colors are used on variable schedules. It has been observed that animals spontaneously seek exposure to colors that feel good to them, and they will avoid colors that feel unpleasant.

Directions: The distance of the light source from the dog should be close enough to expose the entire body of the dog to the colored light, but far enough away from the animal to avoid the heat emitted by the bulb. To test the right distance, place your hand for a short while on your dog's body, allowing the light to expose your hand in the same way it would affect your dog. If the light feels warm, move the light source away until the setup feels pleasant. Use this therapy once or twice daily for approximately five or ten minutes.

Why Combination Remedies?

Original homeopathic treatments consisted solely of single remedies, which means that only single substances were used for any formulation. This method required extraordinary depth of knowledge and understanding of diseases by the health care provider in order to assess the distinct effect of each substance. Such knowledge is based on exceedingly long years of study and experience. In addition, it is important to understand that single remedy formulations at low dilutions will elicit primary aggravating symptoms of disease. This necessary phase of the treatment is difficult to understand for those who have not studied homeopathy in depth.

This book, however, gives the reader the tools and understanding of simple and easy to understand methods and theories that can be used and applied at home. Therefore, single remedies are excluded from the list of suggested home remedies; in their place are a recommended series of homeopathic combination remedies that have proven highly successful.

What Are Combination Remedies?

Combination remedies are formulated by combining a number of single remedies that are all effective for the same disease complex. Combinations of remedies often show their healing effect faster than the single remedies because they reach a larger spectrum of body functions at once. For example, diarrhea is characterized by changes in the consistency and color of the stool. For each variation in consistency and for each possible color change, there are specific single remedies. If you were to use all of them, they would soon overtake your medicine cabinet. In addition, you may not always be able to examine your dog's stool, depending on where the dog relieves itself. In these and other cases you can understand how useful the application of combination remedies is, since the latter are effective in all types of diarrhea.

What was said in the preceding example is true for all other diseases. It is noteworthy, however, that combination remedies can alleviate only the symptoms of a disease and not the underlying cause. If you find that symptoms remain despite your treatment efforts at home, you must take your dog to a veterinarian in order to establish the

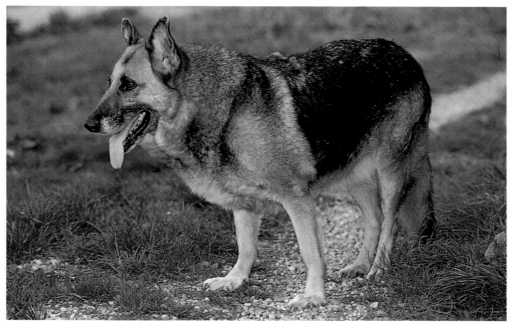

Pet owners can alleviate symptoms of disease in the aging dog by using home remedies.

cause of the disorder. Once a cause is diagnosed, the veterinarian can treat it with specific homeopathic single remedies.

You will find some references in this book that indicate the use of homeopathic single remedies. For your protection these references are limited to medications that are formulated as "Injeel." These are ampules that contain single remedies for oral application. The contents are applied to the mucosal gum surfaces inside the mouth. Because of the specific formulation of these substances, which is referred to as Potentiation Accord, the stage of primary aggravated symptoms is eliminated, and you may use them at home without risking additional problems in your pet.

The effectiveness of home remedies depends on the availability of medications in your local pharmacy. Single remedies may need to be ordered, which delays treatment by several days.

It is important that you consult a veterinarian trained in holistic techniques when you seek the cause of your dog's disease. He is educated and experienced in this particular science and is the only appropriate person to determine the correct single remedy, as well as the appropriate potentiation needed.

Visiting a Veterinarian Trained in Holistic Techniques

It is a good idea to be well-prepared when you plan to take your dog for the first time to a veterinarian trained in holistic techniques. Answer the questions on page 25 at home so that you have all of the information ready when it is needed. Remember that not only are the disorders or symptoms important, but so are the dog's daily environment, general care, nutrition, behavioral patterns, and the psychological adjustment of the dog at this particular time. The entire health and disease history of the dog is equally important. Your dog's health records might point to a problem that has remained from an earlier disorder.

The First Visit

The primary consultation is the foundation for a trusting relationship between the dog, the pet owner, and the health care provider. It is important that the pet owner understand the treatment by the specialist and that the specialist be able to trust the pet owner with correct and consistent administrations of prescribed treatments. Last but not least, the animal must sense the healing intentions of the specialist.

During the primary consultation, which lasts 20–30 minutes, the dog is allowed to move around freely. This makes it easy for the dog to familiarize itself with the strange environment, and to lose its initial fears.

First Exam and Procedures

Following the initial consultation, the dog will undergo a complete physical exam. This exam informs the specialist about the overall symptoms of this animal and about any potential areas of concern. An additional aid in the methodology of diagnosis is the use of bioresonance analysis. This technique was developed in recent years and is based on the principle that the body has its own natural energy field. It is stipulated that an organic disease that manifests itself in the body

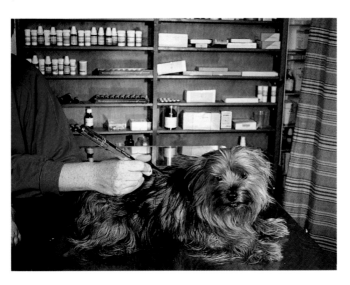

Laser acupuncture painlessly performed on quadruped patients.

Questions for the First Visit

✔ Did you get your dog from a breeder, privately, or from a shelter?

✔ What are the dates of the last vaccinations and last deworming? Were they well tolerated?

✔ Which diseases or surgeries has the dog had?

✔ Has any veterinary clinical diagnosis been made before this visit?

✔ Has the dog been treated? If so, how?

About the home environment:

✔ How do you care for this pet?

✔ What do you feed the pet?

✔ Were there any environmental changes in the dog's life before the current symptoms started?

✔ What is the appearance of the dog's stool, urine, or vomited matter?

✔ Have you noticed changes in the dog's behavior or character?

✔ What are the dog's preferences, e.g., warmth, cold? What does the dog dislike?

result of this test you will receive information not only on the necessary treatment of the disorder under examination but also for any other needs this dog might have at this particular time.

Things to Do After the Initial Diagnosis

A thorough investigation of the causes of a disease will determine not only the type of treatment but also whether or not the disease warrants the use of natural/alternative medicine, or whether veterinary medical treatments are indicated. If you have a good understanding about what is happening inside your animal, you will be able to follow the entire plan of the therapy regimen. The use of home remedies is essential to make the whole of the treatment a success.

must first develop in wavelengths of this energy field. The health care specialist can examine the amplitudes of energy for any incipient points of disease origin with the help of bioresonance analysis.

Using this latest methodology, the veterinarian trained in holistic techniques is able to recognize diseases before they manifest themselves as organic disorders, and he is ready to plan prophylactic treatments before a fulminant disease can develop.

Bioresonance analysis is performed on samples as small as a strand of hair or a drop of blood. As a

How to Locate a Health Care Specialist

The use of the treatments described in this book is mostly referred to as "alternative or holistic medicine," and it is mostly adopted by veterinarians as a complementary option in their treatment specialties. (See Useful Addresses, page 127). If you live in or near a big city, you will have no trouble finding these specialists. In other areas there are many homeopathic and acupuncture practitioners who treat human patients, and who might help you find the indicated prescriptions and formulations.

Symptoms	Causes that Indicate Home Treatment	Warning Signals
Impaired ability to breathe	Foreign body in the throat	1) Inability to breathe following an accident 2) Coughing, 3) Cough, fever, apathy 4) Cough, easily tiring, bluish mucosal surfaces
Cough	Dog got a drop of saliva or food caught in its throat Collar is too tight	1) Itching, watery eyes, nasal discharge 2) Fever, apathy, difficulty breathing 3) Difficulty in swallowing 4) Shortness of breath, bluish mucosals
Itching eyes Itching ears	1) Eye: Sties, see page 35 2) Ear: Eczema, see page 37	1) Watery eyes, caked secretions in the morning 2) Head tilted to one side
Itching skin	Dander, see page 71 Parasites, see page 79 Wrong nutrition	1) Generalized eczema, swelling, reddening, nasal discharge, cough 2) Eczema, hair loss, ear inflammation, dull coat
Staggering, swaying	Normal when dog gets up or shakes head	1) Pale mucosals, slowed pulse 2) Following insect bite 3) Salivation, vomiting, apathy 4) Circling, staring apathetically
Licking	Soiled hair/skin Minor injury	1) Licking genitalia 2) Chewing causing wounds 3) Self mutilation
Salivation	Excitement about females in heat, Car sickness, see page 51 Teething, see page 47 Heartburn, see page 30	1) Vomiting, diarrhea (maybe with blood), lethargy, 2) Staggering, swaying 3) Muscle spasms, thirst but can't drink 4) Mouth odor, swallowing difficulties

Differential Diagnosis   **Description and Treatment**

1) Diaphragmatic rupture, to a veterinary clinic immediately!

2) Enlarged thyroid, tumor, to a veterinary clinic immediately!
3) Bronchitis, lung disorders   3) see pages 40–41
4) Heart disease, to a veterinary clinic immediately!   4) see page 42

1) Allergy   1) see page 72
2) Bronchitis, lung diseases   2) see pages 40–41
3) Tonsillitis   3) see page 51
4) Heart disease, to a veterinary clinic immediately!   4) see page 42

1) Conjunctivitis   1) see page 34

2) Ear inflammations   2) see page 36

1) Allergy
                                                              1) see page 72
2) Liver diseases, kidney disorders, hormonal imbalance
                                                              2) see pages 54, 63

1) Cardiovascular weakness   1) see page 42
2) Allergy   2) see page 72
3) Poisoning   3) see page 95
4) Encephalitis, to a veterinary clinic immediately!

1) Increased sexual drive   1) see page 64
2) Metabolic disorder, to a veterinary clinic immediately!
3) Psychological disturbances   3) see pages 89–91

1) Poisoning   1) see page 95

2) Brain disease, to a veterinary clinic immediately!
3) Infectious diseases, to a veterinary clinic immediately!
4) Gum disease, tonsillitis   4) see pages 48, 51

Symptoms	Causes that Indicate Home Treatment	Warning Signals
Dog drinks excessively	The dog has been very active and playful, he consumes too much food, hot weather	1) Fruit-like mouth odor 2) Urine-like mouth odor, inappetence 3) Vomiting, fever, inappetence 4) Body temperature below normal
Dog drinks too little	Food contains too much moisture	1) Salivation, coughing 2) Salivation, cramps
Dog eats excessively	Dog fasted on previous day, played extensively, does not get enough food	1) Remains thin, hyperactive 2) Fruity smell from mouth, stays thin 3) Continued weight loss, anal area itches, vomiting, diarrhea 4) Drinks much, continues weight loss
Dog eats too little	Unusual food, too hot, too cold, dog ate too much	1) Difficulty swallowing, exhaustion 2) Drinks too much, fever, vomiting, difficulty getting up 3) General malaise, vaginal discharge, lowered temperature 4) Aversion to food, dry and itchy skin, dull coat 5) Salivation, increased thirst, whitish tongue deposits, belching
Vomiting	Dog ate grass, car sickness	1) Itching, reddening, swellings, watering eyes, nasal discharge 2) Diarrhea, inappetence, increased thirst 3) Mucinous stool on thermometer, difficulties eliminating, inappetence 4) Nervousness, choking after eating, stiff gait, belly bloated 5) Salivation, staggering, apathy, blood in stool or secretions

Differential Diagnosis   **Description and Treatment**

1) Diabetes   1) see page 82
2) Kidney disease, uremia, to a veterinary clinic immediately!   2) see page 63
3) Liver disorders, hepatitis, to a veterinary clinic immediately!   3) see page 54
4) Pyometra, to a veterinary clinic immediately!

1) Foreign body lodged in the throat, to a veterinary clinic
   immediately!
2) Paralysis of the pharynx, rabies, to a veterinary clinic
   immediately!

1) Hyperthyroidism, hyperactive hypophysis, to a veterinary clinic
   immediately!
2) Diabetes   2) see pages 81, 82

3) Intestinal parasitism   3) see page 56

4) Pancreatitis,immediately to a veterinary clinic immediately!

1) Gum disease, tonsillitis   1) see pages 48, 51

2) Prostate problems   2) see page 69

3) Pyometra, immediately to a veterinary clinic immediately!

4) Liver diseases   4) see page 54

5) Gastritis   5) see page 53

1) Allergy   1) see page 72

2) Gastrointestinal diseases   2) see pages 51–60

3) Intestinal blockage, to a veterinary clinic immediately!

4) Stomach torsion, to a veterinary clinic immediately!

5) Poisoning   5) see page 95

Symptoms	Potential Causes with Self-Help Indication	Symptoms that Are Warning Signals
Vomiting and fever	May occur as symptom of body's own defense mechanism, purging pathogens	1) Diarrhea, exhaustion 2) Painful urination, moist eczema, exhaustion 3) Dog drinks more, inappetence apathy, itching, dull coat, dehydrated
Heartburn	Food is too soft or bites are too small	Salivation, licking carpets, vomiting food particles
Increased urination	Dog drank too much	1) Dog drinks frequently, fruity smell from mouth, weight loss, vomiting 2) Extreme thirst, general dehydration 3) Moist eczema, fever, exhaustion 4) Painful urination, interrupted urination, bloody urine
Bloating, gas	Unaccustomed food, gas producing ingredients, spoiled food, unadjusted food change	1) Flatus with diarrhea, constipation, gurgling intestinal sounds (growling stomach) 2) Changing stool consistency, (page 111), gray-yellow stool
Diarrhea	Stress, unaccustomed food Food change without adjustment period	1) Alternates with constipation 2) Itching, swelling, reddening, watery eyes, nasal discharge
Diarrhea and vomiting	Stress, unaccustomed food	1) Fever, exhaustion 2) Inappetence, thirst, belching 3) Salivation, apathy, bloody secretions 4) Urinelike smell from mouth, thirst, lack of urination, apathy

Differential Diagnosis	Description and Treatment
1) Parasites 2) Cystitis, nephritis 3) Liver diseases	1) see pages 56, 79 2) see pages 62, 63 3) see page 54
Gastritis	see page 53
1) Diabetes Mellitus 2) Diabetes Insipidus 3) Nephritis 4) Cystitis, bladder stones	1) see page 82 2) see page 81 3) see page 63 4) see page 62
1) Enteritis 2) Pancreatitis, to a veterinary clinic immediately!	1) see pages 57–60
1) Pancreatitis, to a veterinary clinic immediately! 2) Allergy	2) see page 72
1) Parasites 2) Gastritis, gastroenteritis 3) Poisoning 4) Uremia, to a veterinary clinic immediately!	1) see pages 55, 79 2) see pages 51–60 3) see page 95

Treating Diseases at Home

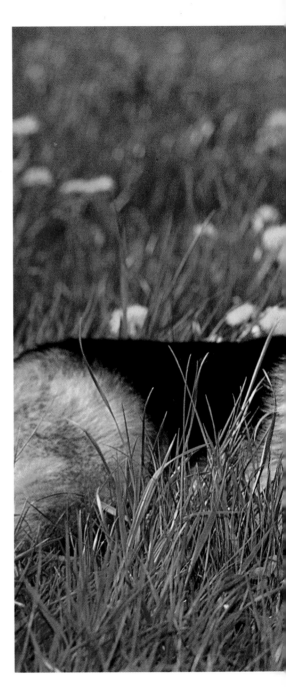

Despite all your best efforts in care and nutrition, you could, one day, find your dog ill.

If you follow the descriptions of diseases and the treatment directions on these pages, you will be able to heal your pet in most cases. Of course, there are exceptions when it is suggested that you seek the advice of a veterinarian trained in holistic techniques. There will be specific instructions for you on how to recognize symptoms of problems that you cannot treat yourself.

For just about all diseases, it can be said that your dog will benefit from certain treatments that will aid or reactivate the process of healing because the immune system and the regenerative powers of the body are damaged by disease.

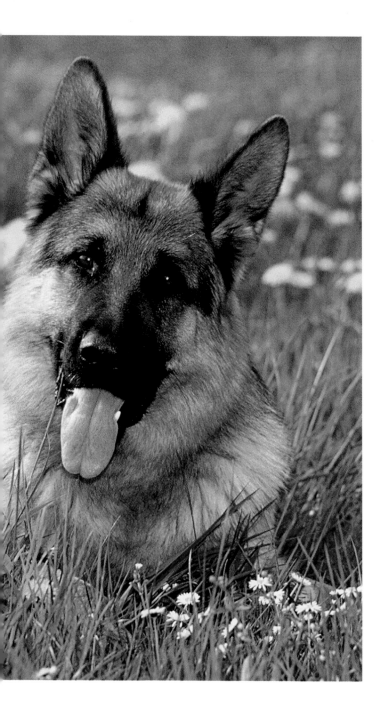

Diseases of the Head and Sensory Organs

Conjunctivitis

If you allow tearing eyes to remain untreated, the condition is bound to develop into a chronic conjunctivitis. This problem is sometimes accompanied by yellowish purulent secretions. As the disease progresses, reddish-brown streaks of tears will mark a line from the corners of the eyes along the nose.

Symptoms
One or both eyes are tearing and the conjunctival lining appears red and swollen. In the morning, you might find the eye caked shut. While the running tears are usually clear, they may or may not be irritating to the surrounding skin. The dog will try to avoid light, and the eyes may be itchy.

If only the left eye is red and runny, you need to consider an underlying kidney disorder.

Causes
There are a number of causes for this disorder: draft, sties, warts, and foreign bodies. Driving in an air-conditioned car may also cause this problem, not to mention allowing your dog to hold its head out of the window of a moving car.

Foreign bodies, such as dust and dirt, are culprits too and so are lashes that are too long and cause irritations. Inflammations of hair follicles can also irritate the conjunctival lining.

In addition, there are causes such as a congenital inversion of an eyelid, allergic reactions, the use of expired, spoiled eyewash solutions, and an inherited condition that causes the constriction or closure of the tear ducts. If a fungal infection is the cause, the eye itself will also become affected.

There are systemic infectious diseases, such as distemper and leptospirosis, which count conjunctivitis as one of their accompanying symptoms. Other diseases of this category are jaundice, anemia, colds, and a number of disorders of the kidneys and the liver.

Self-Help
Important: Never use chamomile or boric acid for the treatment of conjunctivitis. These agents will aggravate the condition.

If you notice that only one eye is affected, pull the lower lid down carefully and inspect it for a loose lash or other foreign body.

● Home Remedies
Use diluted Calendula essence to dab the affected eye carefully, then administer Euphrasia eye drops in both eyes. Treat both eyes because bacterial infections might easily be transmitted from one eye to the other. Follow this treatment by orally giving your dog Keratisal drops. For suggested dosages, see the inside front cover.

When to Consult a Veterinarian
Stop self-help measures when your home remedies do not yield improvement within 3 days or when the white part of the eyes (the sclera) appears either yellowish or pink-yellowish.

What to Expect

The natural therapist (veterinarian trained in holistic techniques) will choose homeopathic remedies that are specifically directed at the problem area. Nosode therapy is designed to eliminate toxins, and cytoplasm therapy may be used in the form of eye drops. There are also specific eye drops that are formulated to act against fungal infections.

Preventive and Convalescent Care

Your dog must be kept away from all drafts. Check the expiration date on your eyewash medications.

Breed Dispositions

Conjunctivitis is frequently encountered in Saint Bernard dogs and in basset hounds.

Sties

These follicular inflammatory enlargements are usually located along the edge of the lid. They can lead to injuries of the cornea and, in some cases, to blindness.

Symptoms

With every reflexive movement of the lid the inflammation is aggravated. This causes the eye to tear and to appear red. In addition, the eye is very itchy.

Causes

Sties are caused by inflammation, secretion, subsequent occlusion, and pus formation of the tiny glands that are found in the eyelid.

Self-Help

Euphrasia drops offer topical relief. Administer one drop every morning and evening. Treat both eyes. These drops *do not irritate* the eyes!

Important: Never use chamomile or boric acid for eye treatments. These agents will further aggravate an already existing inflammation.

● Home Remedies

The medication of choice is Staphisagria-Injeel ampules for oral administration. If after 14 days the condition is not cleared, change to Thuja-Injeel ampules. In case your dog's eyes look red, add oral doses of Belladonna-Injeel ampules. Dosages are listed on the inside front cover. Use diluted Calendula essence to clean caked eye secretions gently from the corners of the eyes.

When to Consult a Veterinarian

If you see no improvement or healing after two weeks of home treatment, you should take your dog for treatments by a specialist.

What to Expect

First, it is necessary to establish the cause of the problem. Could an inherited malformation of the lid be the cause? Once a probable cause is established, the veterinarian trained in holistic techniques can proceed with homeopathic remedies.

If all fails, the dog's sty must be removed by a clinical veterinarian. This procedure is usually performed under local anesthesia. Unfortunately, sties have a habit of recurring.

See page 92 for pre- and postsurgical care.

Preventive and Convalescent Care

If you have one of those dogs who suffers from recurring watery eyes, it would be a good idea to clean the eyes frequently by gently and carefully dabbing Calendula essence on the surrounding areas.

Try to prevent any additional irritations, such as a draft or a very bright sun exposure.

Inflammations of the Ear

Inflammatory ear problems may be part of metabolic disorders or they may be diseases in their own right.

Symptoms

The dog shakes its head over and over again, scratches its ears, tries to slide on its ears along the floor, and/or holds its head tilted at an angle (this is usually indicative of a single ear being affected). All this occurs without any other external signs of disease. Usually the dog will object if you try to touch its ears. Also, if you clean the inner ear, you might find excessive secretions, or even putrid smelling, discolored earwax. Sometimes the condition has progressed to liquefied, brownish deposits containing pus in the ear canal. The same problem may lead to dried, brownish crumbly deposits, which is usually an indication of ear mite infestation.

If this condition is not treated immediately, the problem may affect the inner ear, which will result in a very painful condition. Once it has reached this stage, the dog will not allow anyone to even touch its ears. The pain will induce a dog to bite anyone. In addition, scratching may cause external ear injuries.

Causes

The most common causes of ear problems are parasites, such as ear mites, bacteria, fungal infections, foreign bodies, tumors, and excessive hair growth. Allergic ear reactions may be caused by expired ear cleaning medications.

Inflammatory ear problems, which are restricted to one side only, may be indicative of either foreign bodies that are lodged in the ear canal or they may be expressions of underlying general diseases. For example, left-sided ear inflammations may be indicative of kidney problems or hormonal imbalances, while right-sided ear inflammations may point to nutritional imbalance or to liver function impairment.

Self-Help

Clean the ears with Calendula essence, which you should dilute with boiled or distilled water. Use the directions on page 105. If the ears appear red and hot, use $1/2$ ampule of Traumeel (contains no alcohol and won't burn!) after you have cleaned the ear, and dab it gently on the affected area. Use the remaining $1/2$ ampule for oral administration.

If your dog has pendulous ears, it is a good idea to tape or tie them up on top of the head. This will allow air into the affected areas inside the ear.

Important: Do not use ointments or creams for the treatment of ear problems. These preparations clog the ear, cake up with the additional ear wax, and the original inflammation could get worse.

● Home Remedies

Oral administration of Belladonna-Injeel is indicated for cases where the ears feel hot, appear reddened and are sensitive to the touch. For dogs that are typically heavy and slow and prone to recurring ear problems, the medication of choice is Graphites-Injeel for oral administration.

If the condition has progressed to pus formation, treat your dog once or twice daily with Staphylosal drops. Once the acute inflammation has subsided, give your dog, for a few days, oral doses of Silicea-Injeel. This will enhance the final healing process.

When to Consult a Veterinarian

If an ear inflammation has not improved or healed after one week of your treatment efforts, it is time to see a veterinarian trained in holistic techniques.

What to Expect

First, the veterinarian will establish whether the ear problem is associated with an underlying metabolic disorder. If this turns out to be the case, the dog will receive specific homeopathic medication. If this is not the case, other homeopathic formulations will be chosen to address the local nature of the problem. You will also be instructed in the use of color therapy, so that you can aid the recovery in your home.

Preventive and Convalescent Care

Make it a habit to check your dog's ears daily. In this way, you will find a foreign body or excessive hair growth before they cause serious problems.

Breed Dispositions

Ear problems predominantly affect dog breeds with pendulous ears.

Eczema

Eczematous lesions along the edge of the ear are frequently seen in dogs with floppy ears and in breeds that have their ears cropped.

Symptoms

Eczema usually starts with a simple irritation that itches, whereupon the dog scratches or rubs the affected ear. This insult leads to bleeding and further irritation. While this condition often appears to heal quickly with good scab formation, it might just as quickly be broken by scratching. Subsequently, it can get infected with bacteria or fungi.

Causes

The most common causes are impact, bites, scratching, or continuous shaking of the head. Parasites may also be implicated as causes of eczema.

Self-Help

Treat the affected ear first with diluted Calendula essence, and then follow up by gently rubbing a thin layer of Traumeel ointment on the lesion. Hamamelis ointment is equally suitable.

Important: Try to keep your dog from scratching the affected ear because the scratching will delay the healing process.

When to Consult a Veterinarian

If the edge of the ear remains scabby and bloody despite your treatment efforts, you should seek the help of a professional.

What to Expect

The inflammation will be treated with specific homeopathic remedies. In addition, the process of healing will be aided by the administration of cytoplasm therapy.

Preventive and Convalescent Care

Whenever you examine your dog's ears, include the edges of the ears in your inspection.

Breed Dispositions

Spaniels and basset hounds are affected more frequently than others.

Parotid Gland Inflammation

These glands are located below the ears, just behind the lower jaw.

 Important: Do not mistake these glands for swollen lymph nodes!

Symptoms
Inflammation of these glands appears as marble-sized enlargements just below the ears. The swelling is usually not sensitive to the touch and, at first, only the left side appears to be affected.

Causes
Colds and other viral infections, as well as occlusion of the secretory canal, may be the causes of this condition.

Self-Help
Give your dog one tablet of Traumeel and one ampule of Belladonna-Injeel daily.

Bach Flowers
If your dog appears weakened and tired from the inflammatory condition, administer hornbeam and olive.

When to Consult a Veterinarian
See a professional if your home treatment has not been successful within three days.

Important: If the condition is painful, you should take your dog immediately to a veterinarian trained in holistic techniques.

What to Expect
First, the inflammation will be treated with a specific homeopathic single remedy, which will also stimulate the body's own healing resources. Then, Nosode therapy will be initiated, which will aid the detoxification process. Color therapy may be added to enhance the recovery process.

Preventive and Convalescent Care
Do not expose your dog to drafts.

Diseases of the Respiratory and Circulatory Systems

Nasal Discharge

Most commonly, nasal discharge is part of a cold or flu, but other causes should be considered. This condition should be treated right away in order to prevent secondary problems, such as dry and inflamed nostrils, irritations of the surrounding skin, or sinus infections.

Symptoms

The dog shows watery, nonirritating or irritating nasal discharge. However, the discharge may be thick and puslike, yellowish mucoid, or greenish. A frequent accompanying symptom is the avoidance of light. Sneezing is common, and you will find your dog breathing through its mouth because its nose is clogged with mucus.

Causes

Bacteria, viruses, and fungal infections are the most common causes. Impacted teeth may also cause this condition, and allergies are also often at the root of the problem. Distemper and kennel cough are generalized diseases that are accompanied by nasal discharges.

Important: If the nasal discharge is mixed with blood, you must consider tumors or injuries as a cause. A tumor may also cause a discharge on only one side. These cases should be immediately treated by a health professional.

Self-Help

Euphorbium-comp. oral ampules are indicated for the treatment of nonirritating and greenish yellow discharge. If the nasal discharge is mucoid and stringy, choose Hydrastis-Injeel oral ampules as treatment. Staphylosal drops should be administered in the presence of pus in the discharge. For suggested dosages, see the inside front cover.

When to Consult a Veterinarian

Seek the advice of a veterinarian trained in holistic techniques if your dog gets worse, if it develops a fever, and if you observe blood in the nasal discharge.

What to Expect

Treatments consist mainly of specific homeopathic single remedies that treat the condition and strengthen the body's own defense functions. Nosode therapy will be added to rid the organism of fungal infections or toxins. You will also be instructed in how to use color therapy at home in order to aid in the recovery process.

Preventive and Convalescent Care

Keep your dog away from cold, wet, and drafty places.

Bronchitis, Coughing

A cough can be dry or productive. While coughing is usually associated with disorders of the respiratory system, it is noteworthy that certain diseases of the heart also cause coughing. Bronchitis, an inflammation of the respiratory ducts, is most commonly an acute condition. However, if the disease is not treated in its acute phase, it will progress into a chronic form.

Symptoms

At first, the animal suffers from a dry cough. Eventually, the dog may cough up mucoid and pus-containing sputum. Coughing episodes may be accompanied by shortness of breath, loss of appetite, weakness, unresponsiveness and by fever. If a dog suffers from edema of the lung, the cough will produce a pink foaming sputum, whereas increased pulmonary pressure causes whitish mucoid production. If the condition has progressed to a chronic stage, blood will be coughed up with the inflammatory secretions.

Important: As soon as there is any trace of blood associated with your dog's cough, you should consult a veterinarian. The same goes for signs of pus in the sputum. Foreign bodies, tumors or abscesses may be the causes. Generalized diseases, such as kennel cough or distemper, may also be implicated, especially if the dog appears generally ill.

Causes

The simplest cause for a cough may be a tight collar. Pressure on the throat causes the dog to cough. Other causes of coughing are colds and inflammations of the throat, trachea, or tonsils. The most common causes of bronchitis are bacteria, viruses, and fungi. Then there are tumors, cardiopulmonary disorders, and pleurisy. If the

neck appears swollen, you must also consider thyroid disorders. And if watery eyes and a runny nose are part of the picture, the cause may be an allergic reaction to specific substances in the dog's environment.

Self-Help

Important: Keep your dog quiet and restful, and prevent any exposure to cold, wet, or drafty conditions.

● Home Remedies

If your dog's cough is caused by a regular cold, you may treat the animal daily with Bryaconeel tablets, Cosmochema cough drops, or Tartephedreel drops. If, however, you do not know the cause of the cough, you should use Husteel drops. For dosages, see the inside front cover.

● Bach Flowers

If you find that your dog is weakened and tired from the coughing episodes, treat your pet with hornbeam and olive.

When to Consult a Veterinarian

Seek the advice of a professional if the cough persists more than four days and if your dog's general condition appears to get worse.

What to Expect

Homeopathic single remedies will be administered for the strengthening of the general immune defense system. This will also improve the bronchial and pulmonary tissue functions. Nosodes are used to stimulate the body's ability to purge toxins and bacteria that might have been the causes for the cough.

For regenerative processes, the veterinarian will apply cytoplasm therapy. You will be instructed in the use of color therapy, which will aid the recovery process.

Preventive and Convalescent Care

Your dog's collar or harness should be loose enough to avoid any pressure on the neck. Do not expose your dog to cold and wet weather.

Pneumonia

Pneumonia frequently begins as bronchitis.

Symptoms

Pneumonia is characterized by high fever, apathy, general weakness, tiredness, and a dry cough in the beginning stages. Also, breathing difficulties (especially rapid, labored breathing) and lack of appetite are part of the picture.

Causes

In most cases, we see pneumonia as a consequence or as an accompanying aggravation of a bacterial or viral infection of the lungs. Fungal and parasitic agents may also be the causes.

Dogs that are kenneled outside may contract colds during the winter months, which can develop into pneumonia if they are not recognized early.

Self-Help

Important: A highly nutritious diet will aid the recovery considerably. It should contain meat broth, fresh meats, egg yolks, and some fructose. Add some diluted black tea to your dog's drink menu.

You must see to it that your dog gets absolute "bed rest." The only permitted outings are for the purpose of elimination. It would be best if the dog could rest in a room that gets fresh air without causing a draft.

● Home Remedies

If the fever is higher than 102.2°F (39°C), treat the patient with Febrisal drops. Bryaconeel tablets are indicated for a dry cough. This will also aid the pulmonary function. Use Gripp-Heel tablets to stimulate the body's own defense activities. Suggested dosages are on the inside front cover.

● Bach Flowers

Give your dog crab apple for internal purification. If your patient looks tired or even exhausted, choose hornbeam and olive.

When to Consult a Veterinarian

The fever should be down by the third day and you should see a significant improvement. If this has not occurred, at all cost, take your dog to a veterinarian trained in holistic techniques.

What to Expect

Using specific homeopathic single remedies, the dog will be treated with the goal of strengthening the overall condition of the body and, specifically, the respiratory and circulatory systems. In addition, therapy will include the use of Nosode therapy in order to rid the body of pathogens. You will also be instructed in the application of color therapy to speed the recovery process.

Preventive and Convalescent Care

Protect your dog from exposure to cold, wet, and drafty conditions.

2

Circulatory Impairment

Poor blood circulation may arise as a consequence to a generalized illness, or it may be part of a hereditary disposition.

Symptoms
The dog collapses suddenly and is only minimally responsive. The oral mucosa is pale, the pulse is slowed down or accelerated. As the dog slowly gets up following the episode, you might notice generalized trembling.

Causes
Circulatory disorders may be caused by exertion, heat, or as a sequel to anesthetic or sedative treatments. Infectious diseases, poisoning, or loss of blood from an accident or surgery may also lead to impaired blood circulation.

Self-Help
Quick recognition and immediate first aid are essential when your dog collapses due to heat, exertion, poisoning, or an accident.

Important: Place the animal on a soft surface. Avoid the floor if it is cold. Turn it on its side to prevent aspiration of vomited material. Massage the paws gently in an upward motion in order to stimulate circulation.

● **Home Remedies**
Carbo-vegetabilis-Injeel for oral administration is of immediate help if you carefully place drops on the oral mucosa of your patient. For suggested dosages, see the front inside cover.

● **Bach Flowers**
Rescue drops are highly effective as emergency medication.

When to Consult a Veterinarian
Unless the dog gets better quickly and you see the oral mucosa turn pink soon, you must take your dog for an emergency visit with a veterinarian trained in holistic techniques. The same is true if your dog remains unresponsive and/or if breathing difficulties accompany the collapse.

What to Expect
First, the veterinarian trained in holistic techniques will administer homeopathic single remedies in order to stabilize the cardiovascular system. Subsequently, the priority will be to find an underlying cause for the collapse.

Preventive and Convalescent Care
Keep your dog away from extended exposure to sun and heat. Do not allow exertion during hot summer weather. If you own a dog that has a disposition for circulatory weakness, pre-medicate your animal with Vertigoheel. On potentially critical days, administer one tablet once or twice daily.

Weak Heart

A certain weakness of the heart function may occur after the age of five years. If your dog shows no other generalized health problems, this condition can be controlled by the administration of homeopathic medications.

Symptoms
While the overall health of the dog appears intact, there are indications that your animal tires more quickly, it has lost much of its endurance, and it wants to take a few more snoozes than in earlier years. You might notice that your dog appears out of breath quickly, especially during the summer months. Climbing stairs is beginning to look like a

real effort. If the condition progresses, a dry cough may develop.

Causes

General metabolic functions slow down with age and responsiveness diminishes as well. This initiates stages of organic degenerative processes which in turn lower the capacity of the heart function.

If the dog was trained extensively running next to a bike or performing other sporting activities, it is likely that the animal has developed an enlarged heart, which frequently expresses itself in later years by cardiac weakness.

Self-Help

For an aging dog you must pay close attention to choosing a diet that is easily digestible (see page 14). Too much dry food, like kibbles, should be avoided.

Important: Change your patterns of walking your dog to more frequent and less lengthy outings. While you want to stimulate metabolic activity, you must prevent any exertion.

● Home Remedies

Cralonin-drops and Cactus-comp. drops have proven to be the most reliable and effective medications for the stimulation and strengthening of the cardiovascular system. Also, Cor comp., administered orally once or twice weekly, has proven to have a consistent regenerative effect on the heart.

● Bach Flowers

If your dog is old, tired, and weak, treat it with hornbeam and olive, while cerato should be given to a dog that appears unsteady or overly careful in its movements. Cherry plum is indicated for dogs that panic easily.

When to Consult a Veterinarian

Get professional help when your home treatments remain unsuccessful and if additional symptoms occur.

What to Expect

Homeopathic single remedies will be selected to stimulate and strengthen the general condition of the animal. Subsequently, the dog will receive cytoplasm therapy to effect cardiac regeneration.

Preventive and Convalescent Care

Keep the dog from exerting itself in any way.

Diseases of the Digestive System

Weight Loss

Weight loss can be a normal occurrence in aging dogs, even if the food intake is not reduced. Certain metabolic disorders can also lead to weight loss.

Symptoms
(A) The dog is slender by nature, it is very active, and it has ample play time outdoors.
(B) The animal eats excessively but does not gain weight.
(C) The dog has lost a substantial amount of weight and appears generally ill.

Causes
(A) The dog burns food calories faster than it can eat them.
(B) The following causes must be considered: a hyperactive thyroid gland, pancreatitis, cancer, or a massive parasitic infestation.
(C) A serious metabolic disorder may be the cause.

Self-Help
(A) Increase the amount of food until you can feel but no longer see the ribs of your dog! Do not feed rice because it adds to general loss of fluids.
(B) Have your dog's stool examined for worms. If this turns out negative, you should have the dog checked for a possible metabolic disorder.
(C) This dog belongs in the hands of a veterinarian trained in holistic techniques.

Important: Feed your dog several small meals each day.

● Home Remedies
Orally administer one ampule of Abrotanum-Injeel daily.

● Bach Flowers
If your dog has a strong-willed character, use vine, and if you have a hyperactive, impatient dog, you need to give it vervain or impatiens.

When to Consult a Veterinarian
If your dog has symptoms (B) or (C), you should immediately take your dog to a veterinarian trained in holistic techniques.

What to Expect
The specialist will choose homeopathic single remedies that are targeted at metabolic disorders. The use of Nosode therapy will purge the body of pathogenic organisms. In some cases, the use of cytoplasm therapy may be indicated in order to stimulate the body's regenerative abilities. Acupuncture might also be used to free blocked meridians. You will be instructed in the use of color therapy to aid the recovery process in your home. Acupressure may also be indicated for home use.

Preventive and Convalescent Care
Optimal nutrition is the most important preventive measure you can take (see page 14).

Breed Dispositions

Many breeds are naturally "thin," especially the borzoi, pinscher, and whippet.

Obesity, Potbelly

In cases of obesity, one has to distinguish between overall fat and localized, abnormal fat, such as a fat belly. Metabolic disorders will show up more readily in fat animals than normal weight animals. Fat dogs are also more inclined to suffer from musculo-skeletal problems, cardiovascular disorders, and respiratory impairments.

Symptoms

(A) The dog increases in weight by putting on fat all over its body.
(B) Despite a well-balanced and restricted meal plan, the dog is roly-poly from puppyhood on.
(C) The animal is getting rounder without increasing its food amount. The animal appears slow or lethargic.
(D) The dog's belly is getting rounder, while the rest of the body remains unchanged.
(E) Following neutering, i.e., spaying or castration, dogs tend to put on weight.

Causes

(A) You are feeding your dog too much. Maybe your dog does not get enough outdoor activity to burn the food calories.
(B) You probably have a dog with a congenital disposition of obesity (see page 120).
(C) The cause could be an underproduction of thyroid hormone.
(D) Too much food is usually the cause of a potbelly. Could the dog be pregnant? A pyometra must

also be considered, as well as ascites, a tumor, a gastric torsion, liver and spleen enlargements, or Cushings disease.
(E) Neutered dogs slow their activities but not their hunger.

Self-Help

(A) Reduce the amount of food and increase activities.
(B), (C), (D) Seek a diagnosis from a veterinarian trained in holistic techniques.
(E) In neutered animals, it may be necessary to develop a homeopathic treatment plan that affects the overall constitution of the dog. A specialist will have to create specific treatment combinations for each case.

● **Bach Flowers**

This therapy will be indicated only if your dog shows symptoms of psychological disorders. If you are dealing with a strongly dominant animal, choose vine as treatment. For nervous, fearful, or shy dogs, get mimulus, and if jealousy is apparent, use holly.

When to Consult a Veterinarian

Take your dog to a veterinarian trained in holistic techniques if you are sure that your dog is not pregnant and that you are not overfeeding your pet. Do go, also, if you notice other symptoms that appear to affect the general well-being of your dog.

What to Expect

Depending on each particular case history, the treatment may involve homeopathic medications to regulate metabolic disorders, cytoplasm therapy to regenerate damaged cell systems, or the use of Nosodes to detoxify the body.

3

Preventive and Convalescent Care

Priority must be given to an optimal nutrition plan (see page 14).

If your dog tends to overeat and is inclined to beg, you are better off feeding several small meals each day.

If your dog is naturally plump, you should add rice to the food because it will reduce water retention.

Make sure that your dog gets ample time for walks and physical activities.

Breed Dispositions

Obesity affects dachshund and spaniel dogs more than other breeds.

Swallowing Disorders

Impairment of the ability to swallow is frequently the reason why a dog that is normally a good eater suddenly refuses food. It is important that the owner observe and keep track of a dog's eating patterns.

Symptoms

You can tell that the dog is hungry as it approaches the food bowl, but instead of eating, the dog lies down next to the food. If someone approaches, the dog will defend its food, yet will not eat it.

Other symptoms are: increased salivation, swallowing without food intake, clearing the throat or coughing, and very slow or careful water intake.

The throat is usually found to be red and inflamed. Fever, weakness, and frequent yawning may also be observed.

Causes

Inflammations of the pharynx, larynx, tonsils, and the trachea, as well as of the esophagus, are the most common causes that lead to an impairment in swallowing.

Other causes are food that is too hot, eating snow, persistent barking, chronic heartburn, or injuries. A collar that is too tight, as well as the habit of pulling on a leash while walking, are also conditions that lead to impairment of swallowing because of the pressure that is exerted on the neck.

Other causes that have to be distinguished are insect bites, injuries of the palate, or the existence of a congenital cleft palate.

If the general health appears to be affected at the same time the swallowing difficulties are observed, foreign bodies, tumors, abscesses in the throat area, nerve damage, or an enlarged thyroid could be at the root of the problem.

Important: Some infectious diseases are associated with swallowing difficulties. These are rabies, leptospirosis and hepatitis. Seek the advice of a veterinarian trained in holistic techniques if you are not sure of the cause of your dog's problems.

Self-Help

Using care not to be bitten, check the mouth and throat for foreign bodies, and remove any that might be lodged there. Check for insect stings and any type of injuries. Check the collar and loosen it if necessary. If all mechanical causes can be excluded, there is usually an inflammatory process at the root of the problem.

Note: Depending on your dog's temperament, you may want to ask someone to assist you in examining the animal's mouth and throat.

● Home Remedies

During the first two to three days, administer Arconitum-Injeel ampules orally. If swallowing is not fully back to normal after three days, you can aid the body's detoxification process by giving your dog Lymphomyosot drops. In addition, you can speed the healing of the mucosal surfaces of the mouth by administering Mucosa comp. drops orally.

For suggested dosages, see the front inside cover.

If you can, instill some diluted sage tea. Most dogs will not accept this application because the flavor of the tea is too strong.

● **Bach Flowers**

To enhance the detoxification process, you should give your dog crab apple. In addition, you may use hornbeam in case your pet is listless and lethargic due to its swallowing problems.

When to Consult a Veterinarian

Consult a veterinarian trained in holistic techniques if your treatments have not been successful within three days, or if additional symptoms occur.

What to Expect

First, the overall constitutional condition will be strengthened with the help of classic homeopathic remedies.

If the problem is caused by organic disease, the dog will receive specific single remedies. Nosode therapy is indicated if the specialist finds toxins at the root of the disorder.

Preventive and Convalescent Care

Make sure the collar is not too tight and train your dog not to pull on the leash.

Regular vaccination boosters are necessary to prevent infectious diseases.

Do not allow your dog to eat snow, and keep your dog away from cold and wet environments. Water puddles are full of bacteria and other agents, and they should be off-limits to your dog.

Hot food is not suitable for your dog. Keep the temperature moderately warm. Optimal nutrition

(see page 14) prevents heartburn. The latter may irritate the throat because stomach acid flows back up and burns the lining of the throat.

Toys must be selected according to the size of your dog. Watch out for parts or pieces that can be swallowed and get stuck in the throat.

Breed Dispositions

Swallowing disorders can occur in all breed as a symptom of colds. Increased incidents have been observed in boxers and in American Eskimo dogs. They are commonly caused by inflammation of the pharynx, larynx, trachea, or esophagus.

Teething Problems

Dogs change their dentition between the fourth and sixth month of age. In some animals all goes smoothly, while in others you encounter inflammation and pain.

Symptoms

The gums may turn bright red, there is usually increased salivation, and sometimes the dog will be very sensitive to touch in the mouth area. If you allow the condition to proceed untreated, it is likely that the dog will suffer recurring gingivitis for the rest of its life.

Causes

One cause may be a congenital defect of the outer layer of the teeth. Another cause could be a case of undiagnosed early age distemper that results in teething problems a few months later.

Milk teeth that do not fall out are also likely causes of teething problems. Remaining milk teeth must be removed surgically.

Self-Help

Important: Avoid exertion and hard play during the teething phase. Your dog is more susceptible to problems now.

● Home Remedies

The development of a healthy dentition can be aided by oral administration of one tablet of Calcium fluoratum C30 twice each week. If the gums are inflamed, treat your dog with oral ampules of Belladonna-Injeel.

● Bach Flowers

The use of walnut would be indicated if your dog is undergoing teething problems at the same time it is changing environments, has a new owner, or is removed from its mother.

Choose hornbeam if the teething problem leaves the animal tired and listless, but use vervain for the dogs that react with hyperactivity.

When to Consult a Veterinarian

Consult a veterinarian trained in holistic techniques if your home treatments do not noticeably reduce the inflammation.

What to Expect

In order to improve the body's mineral metabolism, the veterinarian will administer homeopathic single substance medications.

Persistent milk teeth must be removed under anesthesia by a veterinarian.

Gum Disease

This problem develops slowly and often goes unnoticed until it has become a chronic condition. It is therefore important to inspect your dog's mouth, teeth, and gums regularly.

Symptoms

During your routine inspection of your dog's mouth, you will notice that the edges of the gums are quite red. There also may be swelling and bleeding.

Bad mouth odors commonly accompany this condition.

Sometimes the dog will drink water but refuse food.

Tumors, blisters, and thrush (see page 122) can be identified by the changes in the mucosal surfaces as long as these problems are not located way back in the jaws. The edges of the gums appear red and swollen. The swelling may be so severe that it forms a cauliflowerlike enlargement of the gum tissue.

Causes

Gum disease may be caused by injuries, a bad tooth, tartar deposits, or infections with bacteria, viruses, or fungi.

Inflammation may also occur as a consequence of diabetes or uremia.

Left untreated, gum disease can progress to abnormal growths of the gum tissue and lead to heart disease.

Self-Help

Important: Do not forget that cleaning your dog's teeth should be part of your routine pet care (see page 105). Do not give your dog bones to chew on during this period. Bones could increase irritation and injury.

Dab the affected gums with a solution of Dental-Can, or with diluted Calendula essence. In addition, administer one ampule of Belladonna-Injeel daily. Melaleuka-solution has also proven to be highly effective. While this medication won't burn the mucosals, it has a rather strong smell and, for this reason, is usually forcefully rejected by dogs.

● Home Remedies

Oral administration of Phytolacca-Injeel ampules and of Traumeel tablets has proven most effective for the treatment of painful gums. Because Traumeel does not burn, you can dab the gums with it. To do this, use a cotton swab and drop the medication on the swab while dabbing the affected area.

If you notice a foul odor from the mouth, give your dog either Kreosot-Injeel or Mercurius-Injeel orally.

● Bach Flowers

Hornbeam and mustard are good choices if your pet is generally exhausted and listless because of its gum disease.

When to Consult a Veterinarian

Consult a veterinarian trained in holistic techniques if more symptoms appear or if your treatment efforts remain ineffective.

What to Expect

First, the holistic veterinarian will establish whether a bad tooth has caused the problem. If this is the case, the veterinarian will extract the tooth under anesthesia. You will receive the appropriate medications and instructions for pre- and postsurgical care of your patient.

For the improvement of the overall health condition, as well as for the treatment of metabolic disorders, your dog will receive specific homeopathic remedies. Nosode therapy will be employed to purge the body of toxins. Dental deposits will be removed.

Preventive and Convalescent Care

Check your dog's teeth and clean them regularly.

Breed Dispositions

Miniature breeds show more gum disease than others.

Tartar

About 80 percent of all dogs suffer from tartar deposits on their teeth some time during their lives.

If not attended to, tartar can lead to such serious conditions as heart disease.

Symptoms

There are whitish, or yellow-brown mineral deposits at the base of the teeth. These deposits push underneath the gum tissue, which in turn reacts with inflammation, odor, and periodontal disease.

Causes

Tartar is mainly a sign of poor tooth care. Food remnants stay lodged and harden until they become mineralized deposits. Incorrect nutrition and finely minced food particles may also cause this problem. In addition, there is a hereditary condition that predisposes animals to chronic tartar.

Important: Remember to clean your dog's teeth regularly! (See page 105.)

If you get in the habit of giving your dog a hard dog biscuit every night, there is less chance for food remnants to hide between the teeth. Veal bones also do a good job from time to time. No bones, however, for dogs who suffer from recurring constipation. Once you see that tartar is already accumulated, try to scrape it off with your fingernail. This will only work if the material is not yet too old and mineralized.

When to Consult a Veterinarian

Leave the removal of heavy and old deposits to a specialist. The same goes for evidence of red and swollen gums.

3

What to Expect

More often than not, it will take an anesthetic procedure to get rid of the tartar thoroughly. In addition, you can use prescribed homeopathic single remedies that are formulated to generate a healthy dentition.

Preventive and Convalescent Care

Turn to page 105 for advice on cleaning your dog's teeth.

Offer your dog the best nutrition you possibly can (see page 14).

Remember the nightly biscuits.

Do not cut meats into tiny bits.

If the gum line looks inflamed, dab the surface with Dental-Can solution.

Mouth Odors

The majority of cases are caused by dental tartar. Metabolic disorders, however, could cause similar problems.

Symptoms

The dog's breath has a very unpleasant odor. The type of odor depends on the cause (see chart on this page). The animal shows no interest in food because there are either painful areas inside the mouth or the animal is suffering from severe metabolic or organic disorders.

Causes

There are a number of causes for bad mouth odors, each of which may be diagnosed by specific characteristics.

If the cause is	The mouth smells
Tartar, gum disease	putrid
Inflammation	putrid
Abscessed tooth	putrid
Tonsillitis	putrid
Kidney disorders	urinelike
Diabetes	fruity
Oral tumors	rotting

Other accompanying symptoms may turn up. If the cause is not diagnosed and treated, it is likely that inflammatory conditions will get worse and turn into serious disease like uremia or a diabetic coma.

Self-Help

Important: If you find that the odor smells fruity, which may indicate diabetes, rush your dog to a veterinarian trained in holistic techniques. *Do not try home remedies!* The same holds true if your dog's mouth has a urinelike odor (which may indicate kidney disorders).

Avoid the use of any treatments in the form of drops, because they will hurt your animal. Drops are formulated with alcohol, which will burn an inflamed mucosal surface.

If you are clearly dealing with a case of dental deposits, see page 49. If the gums are red and inflamed, see page 48.

When to Consult a Veterinarian

Mouth odors that smell fruity or urinelike must be treated professionally right away. Other mouth odors may be treated with home remedies. If your home treatments are not effective you need to consult a veterinarian trained in holistic techniques.

What to Expect

Metabolic disorders and a weak immune system are best reenergized and regulated with classic homeopathic single remedies. Toxins will be eliminated through the application of Nosode therapy.

Preventive and Convalescent Care

If you remember to give your dog a nightly dog biscuit, you will not only be rewarded with true love but with less dental tartar problems. Check your dog's mouth from time to time, so that you find deposits in their beginning stages. You will also locate small inflammatory areas before they get infected and turn into serious health problems.

Tonsillitis

This disease affects both the very young and the older dogs.

Symptoms

Tonsillitis is commonly first noticed when the dog appears to have difficulties swallowing. The dog acts tentative when it wants to drink or eat. Other symptoms are yawning, increased salivation, bad mouth odor, and attempts by the animal to scratch its throat. The dog becomes unresponsive to invitations for play. The body temperature may rise to 104°F (40°C) and cause the animal to become lethargic and drowsy.

Causes

Tonsillitis can be caused by bacteria, or it can occur as a secondary infection with viral diseases.

Self–Help

Allow your pet absolute rest! Outings are solely for the purpose of elimination.

● Home Remedies

Administer Lymphomyosot drops. If the temperature exceeds 102.2°F (39°C), add Febrisal drops. For suggested dosages, see the inside front cover.

● Bach Flowers

If the animal appears listless and depressed, treat it with hornbeam.

When to Conult a Veterinarian

Get help from a veterinarian if symptoms and fever have not regressed after three days.

What to Expect

Homeopathic remedies will be used to reduce the inflammatory condition and to stimulate the body's own defense mechanisms.

Nosode therapy will be employed in order to eliminate specific toxins.

You will be asked to apply color therapy in order to support the healing process.

Preventive and Convalescent Care

Do not offer your dog ice cold water, and do not allow the animal to drink from street puddles.

Vomiting

When your dog eats grass or accumulates hair in the stomach, vomiting occurs as a kind of physiological purging. If, however, the vomiting occurs repeatedly, there is usually an illness responsible. In this case the cause must be diagnosed.

Important: During prolonged vomiting episodes the body loses a lot of fluids, which often causes circulatory problems and mineral deficiencies. See to it that your pet replenishes the loss with plenty of fresh drinking water.

3

Symptoms

The dog regurgitates its stomach contents. The animal is most likely seen standing stiffly, with its neck stretched out.

(A) Food or liquid (e.g., milk) is thrown up almost as fast as it was swallowed. In some cases the animal will eat its vomited material right away.

(B) The dog vomits while riding in a car.

(C) The vomited matter smells like garlic.

(D) The vomit is tinged with light red blood.

(E) The dog vomits mostly early in the mornings, prior to eating. The vomit is light yellow mucoid.

It is essential that you record the time when the vomiting occurs and the color and consistency of the vomited material.

Important: If vomiting occurs simultaneously with unsuccessful attemps to defecate, there is a serious possibility of an underlying stomach torsion. Take the animal immediately to an emergency clinic! A surgical correction must be performed as soon as possible.

Causes

(A) The dog ate too fast. Throwing up milk or medications may indicate an intolerance to these substances. Vomiting may also indicate an attempt by the body to rid itself of toxins, such as spoiled foods.

(B) The dog is carsick, or it is afraid of riding in a car. Psychological stress may well be part of the cause.

(C) Garlic odor points in the direction of poisoning with phosphorus from ingesting rat poison or insect killing chemicals.

(D) Blood in the vomit usually stems from injuries inside the mouth caused by foreign bodies, such as bone splinters sticking in the pharynx or in the esophagus.

(E) Yellow mucoid vomit is mainly caused by metabolic disorders of the liver and gall bladder in combination with gastritis.

Other causes for vomiting may be serious organ disease, such as pyometra, uremia, jaundice, intestinal occlusion, poisoning, brain contusions, or kidney disorders. In addition, there are inflammations of the mouth and pharynx, tumors, ulcers, pancreatic and adrenal diseases, as well as diabetes.

Vomiting may also be one of several accompanying symptoms of infectious diseases, such as distemper or parvo virus infection, and of heavy worm infestation.

Bitches can also be observed vomiting while they are pregnant or pseudopregnant.

Self-Help

Important: In cases with symptoms (C) and (D) you must take the animal to a veterinary clinic immediately! Do so, also, if a stomach torsion is suspected!

In all other cases, get your pet started on a specific diet for digestive disorders (see page 106). Do not make any physical demands on your animal at this time.

For car sickness administer Rescue drops approximately 30 minutes before you get into the car. Also add Cocculus-Hcc. Use 5–10 drops of each medication. If necessary, you can repeat the medication during a prolonged drive.

● **Home Remedies**

Give Vomisal drops and Gastricumeel tablets. For dosages, see the inside front cover.

● **Bach Flowers**

By giving your dog crab apple you can enhance the effect of the treatment. If the patient is tired and depressed, add hornbeam.

When to Consult a Veterinarian

Get help if vomiting continues after two days, or if car sickness continues after the third trip despite treatment.

Important: It is suggested that you consult a veterinarian trained in holistic techniques if other symptoms occur, such as fever, inappetence, diarrhea, constipation, traces of blood, or a typical garlic odor.

What to Expect

The underlying cause will be diagnosed, and you may be referred to a veterinary specialist for further treatment.

Should this not be necessary, homeopathic single remedies will be employed in order to regulate metabolic pathways and to improve the general condition of the dog. Nosode therapy may be considered for the elimination of toxins.

You will be asked to aid the healing process by applying color therapy at home.

For dogs suffering from car sickness, the veterinarian will prescibe a mild herbal product that calms the dog without dulling it, and that has no side effects.

Preventive and Convalescent Care

Make sure that your dog is left in peace and without interruptions while it is eating. In order to care for the recovering dog, administer Mucosa comp. ampules orally twice a week. This will heal the mucosal linings of the affected digestive organs.

Do not feed your dog when you have to take it for a drive! You can get your dog used to car travel by taking it on short drives, and by taking the animal during the training phase only to places where it associates good memories with a previous visit.

Gastritis

Gastritis is an inflammation of the lining of the stomach. It is one of the most common digestive problems of dogs.

Symptoms

The dog vomits yellow mucous material without evidence of food remnants.

While the general well-being of the dog does not appear to be affected, there may be reduced appetite.

The animal is seen eating more grass than normal, and belching is more frequent.

In addition, the tongue may show a dirty gray layer, thirst is increased, so is salivation, and trembling is not uncommon.

If diarrhea and vomiting appear regularly over an extended period, it can be assumed that a chronic stomach problem exists.

Causes

Frequently diagnosed causes of gastritis are spoiled food, poisoning, stress, or toxic impact on the gastric mucosa.

Winter brings another cause, that of eating snow.

Food that is too hot or too cold, as well as access to chemicals, can also cause gastritis.

Gastritis can also be a symptom that is part of another disease, for example congestive heart failure, liver disorders, or infectious diseases such as distemper or Leptospirosis. Uremic disease may also be accompanied by gastritis.

When dogs lick inflamed wounds containing pus the gastric mucosa can also become irritated.

Self-Help

Prevent your dog from licking chemicals or infected wounds.

Check the expiration dates of foods and medications.

Make sure that your dog gets plenty of rest after running and rough play.

Do not allow your dog to eat snow.

Check the temperature of the food you are feeding your dog. Prepare a specific diet (see page 106).

Important: Try to prevent any stress for your dog at this time!

● Home Remedies

You can give your dog either Gastricumeel tablets or Cosmochema gastrointestinal drops. As soon as the symptoms recede, give your patient mucosa comp. ampules orally.

● Bach Flowers

If your animal appears depressed or sad due to its illness, you can revitalize it with hornbeam and mustard. To enhance internal cleansing, give the dog crab apple.

When to Consult a Veterinarian

If the condition has not responded to your treatment after two or three days you should get the underlying cause evaluated and diagnosed by a veterinarian trained in holistic techniques.

What to Expect

Homeopathic remedies will reestablish a normal physiological stomach function, while the use of Nosodes will aid in the elimination of toxins. You will be asked to continue home treatments by using color therapy.

Preventive and Convalescent Care

Increase the amount of fresh foods and check the temperature of your dog's meals to make sure that they are neither too hot nor too cold.

Check your home thoroughly to make sure that your dog has no access to any chemicals.

Breed Dispositions

Most miniature breeds are predisposed to hypersensitive stomach function.

Liver Disorders

The liver is the Grand Central Terminal for metabolic pathways and for detoxification processes. This means that there is a good chance that some liver disorder might occur in any dog's life.

Important: The main alarm signal for liver disorders is the color yellow. The mucosal surfaces (e.g., the gums) usually turn to a yellow tinge first.

Symptoms

A lack of appetite is usually the first sign of trouble. You might see the dog standing in front of the food bowl, but soon the animal will turn away as if the food looked distasteful.

Another characteristic of animals with liver disorders is the strange pattern of eating at night. This is because the liver is no longer able to follow a normal physiologic pattern of metabolic and detoxifying functions.

The body searches for other ways to get rid of the toxins. Skin and ears are then called upon to assist. That is the reason why a liver disorder is often accompanied by dry eczema, itching, dandruff, and otitis. The otitis usually begins on the right side only, and is followed by dark colored urine. Subsequently, the stool turns light gray-yellow and takes on a claylike consistency. Vomiting yellow foam follows, accompanied by weakness, depression, and apathy.

Important: Take your dog to a veterinarian trained in holistic techniques as soon as you notice that the white of the eyes gets a yellowish tinge. This is a sign of advanced liver disease.

Causes

All types of toxins can cause liver diease. They accumulate there because the liver is supposed to detoxify everything your dog eats. Chemical preservatives are part of this group.

Other causes for liver disease are metabolic disorders in the processing of proteins, carbohydrates, or fats.

Severe infectious diseases, advanced cardiac disease, or massive worm infestation can also lead to liver disease.

Self-Help

The best way to unburden the liver is through a specific diet (see page 106). Start feeding the diet as soon as you notice the discoloration of the stool. If you have an older dog, you might as well keep the animal on this diet forever. If your dog is young, the veterinarian will advise you on the duration of the diet schedule.

Important: Eliminate any and all spicy or fatty foods from your dog's menu. Absolutely no chocolate either!

● **Home Remedies**

For the improvement of liver function the following medications are indicated: Hepeel tablets, Lycopodium-Injeel ampules, Cosmochema liver-gall bladder drops, or Flor de Piedra D12 tablets. Chelidonium-Injeel ampules are suggested if inappetence, vomiting, and gray stools are prominent symptoms. For suggested dosages, see the front inside cover.

● **Bach Flowers**

Do give your dog crab apple before you do anything else. In addition, you may choose from vine or water violet if your patient appears grumpy or unresponsive. If, however, your pet is aggressive or behaves irritably administer beech and holly. The weak and listless pet needs holly and hornbeam.

When to Consult a Veterinarian

It is most useful to consult a veterinarian trained in holistic techniques as soon as you notice a marked change in your dog's eating pattern, because an early understanding of the cause can prevent serious disease.

What to Expect

Homeopathic single remedies will be selected in order to regulate liver function and basic metabolic pathways.

Cytoplasm therapy will be used in an effort to stimulate the regenerative abilities of damaged liver cells.

You will be instructed in the use of color therapy in order to assist the recovery process at home.

Preventive and Convalescent Care

The most appropriate way to prevent liver disorders is a good diet (see page 14). During the recovery period you can assist with one to two oral administrations of Hepar-comp. ampules.

3

Intestinal Parasites (Endoparasites)

There are a number of parasites. Most of them are worm parasites, such as tapeworm, roundworm, hookworm, and whipworm.

Symptoms

Endoparasites cause anal itching. This itch causes the dog to bite its tail or slide on its hindquarters along the floor, which in turn causes inflammation of the anal area.

Depending on the type of worm infestation, symptoms may vary:

(A) The dog loses weight despite regular meals and a healthy appetite. Diarrhea occurs sporadically. Around the anal orifice and in the stool will be 5–10 mm rectangular shaped white organisms sometimes in small clumps like rice grains.

(B) The dog appears emaciated despite normal food intake. Diarrhea, flatulance, and vomiting occur. As the infestation progresses, bronchitis or pneumonia may develop. White worms approximately 10–15 cm long are found in the stool.

(C) The dog has pale mucosals and diarrhea tinged with blood.

(D) The dog is very weak. If diarrhea develops, it usually contains blood.

Causes

(A) Tapeworm infestation is the cause. This parasite is transmitted through the ingestion of infested meats, rats or mice, and fleas.

(B) Roundworms are contracted by ingesting uncooked meats or exposure to infected fecal matter. These parasites live in the small intestine from where they can migrate to the lungs and cause bronchitis and pneumonia.

(C) Hookworms are the cause here. They live in the small intestine where they attach to the lining and suck blood.

(D) Whipworms are the cause. They are found in the stool.

While many parasites are transmitted by the ingestion of raw meats, your dog can also pick up endoparasites during its daily walks because other dogs leave their excrements ready to be sniffed at.

Self-Help

Important: Make it a habit to get your dog's stool analyzed twice each year. Depending on the degree of infestation you can treat your dog biologically or, if the problem is severe, you can use a chemical worm treatment.

Do not use any worm treatment if there is no indication of worms or worm eggs. Such unnecessary treatment would only burden your dog's general metabolic functions.

● Home Remedies

Administer Tanacet-Heel for ten days, 1–3 times daily, 5–10 drops each time. Follow with oral administrations of Mucosa comp., twice a week for two weeks.

● Bach Flowers

If the dog requires worm treatment, you can use crab apple to assist the effectiveness of the medication.

When to Consult a Veterinarian

As soon as you suspect endoparasites you should get the dog's stool analyzed. If it turns out that worms are not the cause and you have treated your dog unsuccessfully for diarrhea or vomiting, you will need to consult a veterinarian trained in holistic techniques in order to establish the cause of the illness.

What to Expect

If a worm infestation is confirmed, the veterinarian trained in holistic techniques will treat your dog with a prescribed biological medication. In addition, the immune system will be stimulated through the administration of homeopathic remedies that enhance overall constitutional strength. This will discourage any future parasitic invasion.

Preventive and Convalescent Care

Have your dog's stool checked for worms twice each year!

Always deep freeze all meats before you cook them for your dog.

Keep an eye on your dog while walking outdoors to prevent him from ingesting any inappropriate material.

Diarrhea

Diarrhea is not a disease in itself, but it is rather a symptom of a disorder in your dog. It is one of the most common symptoms of trouble that you will encounter in a dog's life. Pups and young dogs are especially susceptible to changes in their environment and quickly react with diarrhea.

In most cases it can be said that diarrhea is the body's way of trying to get rid of unwelcome substances.

Important: If the dog has not resumed normal stool formation within three days after a diarrhea incident, you should consult a veterinarian. Serious metabolic disorders may develop or they may be the underlying cause of the problem.

Symptoms

Diarrhea is characterized by a change in the consistency of the stool. It may appear watery, foaming, slimy, or thick and sticky, or it may contain undigested food particles.

The color could be anything from colorless to light clay, yellow, dark, or even black. Blood may also be present.

You must pay close attention to the color, consistency, and odor of the stool. These observations are essential for a health care provider when a treatment becomes necessary.

Sometimes the dog will experience pain when defecating.

Diarrhea is frequently accompanied by a lack of thirst and appetite, or by the opposite symptoms, increased thirst and appetite.

Vomiting and fever are also often observed. Loss of fluids causes the dog to become dehydrated and weak, leading to listlessness and apathy.

Repeated episodes of diarrhea lead to weight loss, dull hair coat, and a general poor appearance.

Causes

The majority of diarrhea incidents are caused by incorrect diets: too many dairy products, too many new foods, a quick change of food types, or exclusively dry or canned foods.

If the dog is fed a commercial diet, it may be possible that the diarrhea is a reaction to certain chemical preservatitives in the currently consumed food type.

Diarrhea can also be caused by stress, and by excitement, such as joy, anger, sadness, spite, shock, fear, or physical exertion. In addition, diarrhea may develop as part of a cold or an infectious disease.

When symptoms of diarrhea and constipation seem to take turns, the cause may be a disorder of the pancreas or a lack of digestive enzymes. Such cases should be seen by a veterinarian as soon as possible.

3

Self-Help

On the first day of the symptomatic episode do not feed your dog. Offer only water.

On the second day you need to begin feeding a strict diet that is formulated for digestive disorders (see page 106). Continue this diet until the stool maintains normal consistency.

It is important that you do not exert your dog during this time, and that you keep the animal cool during hot summer weather.

Important: Do not give your dog charcoal tablets. This will block its natural absorptive abilities, as well as the body's own detoxification processes.

Make sure that your pet drinks sufficient amounts of fresh water to prevent circulatory problems, as well as mineral losses. Thin black tea is a good supplement. If your dog does not like to drink it, use a syringe to administer the tea right into the mouth (see page 102).

● Home Remedies

If you are dealing with a watery type of diarrhea, give your dog one or two capsules of Perenterol daily until the stool appears normal. Diarrheel tablets, once every half hour, are indicated if the stool is mucoid or soft. Use five Cho Dysenteral drops twice a day if the diarrhea looks like rice water.

● Bach Flowers

Crab apple, at a dose of five drops three times a day is indicated for all types of diarrhea. Sometimes the diarrhea is accompanied by behavioral problems.

If the dog acts	Administer
Fearful, nervous, trembling	Aspen
Disinterested, listless	Clematis
Tired, exhausted	Hornbeam
Exhausted, weak	Olive
Apathetic	Wild rose

When to Consult a Veterinarian

A case of diarrhea that has lasted longer than three days should be seen by a veterinarian.

Important: Take your dog to a veterinary clinic immediately if there is blood in the stool, or if the dog vomits foamy or blood tinged material. These symptoms may be caused by poisoning.

What to Expect

A veterinarian trained in holistic techniques will prescibe a homeopathic single remedy that is directed at the specific cause of the diarrhea and that will also strengthen the circulation. Nosode therapy will be employed in order to rid the body of disease causing toxins.

Preventive and Convalescent Care

The most reliable preventive measure for diarrhea is a balanced diet (see page 14). Have a stool exam done twice annually (see page 8).

Do not allow your dog to drink from street puddles.

If the diarrhea was caused by an incorrect diet, you should not try to change everything overnight. Doing this might aggravate the condition, and you will not know if it was caused by the new food.

Treat your dog gently, and avoid physical and psychological exertions. Once the stool has returned to normal consistency, it is best to feed several small meals that are low in meats until the intestinal flora has reestablished itself to normal levels.

You can aid the regeneration of the intestinal mucosa by giving your dog Mucosa comp. orally at a dose of $1/2$ ampule every other day.

Constipation

Constipation is caused more frequently than not by hardening of the stool. There are only rare cases where defecation is inhibited despite a soft stool consistency.

Symptoms
The dog eliminates little or no formed stool.

The elimination may be accompanied by whining because of painful straining.

The animal attempts to defecate repeatedly, but unsuccessfully.

If left untreated, the condition can last for days.

Once in a while there may be evidence of a few drops of thin stool, either foamy or mixed with blood. This must not be mistaken for diarrhea! (see page 57).

The abdomen could appear ballooned and very hard to the touch due to the constipated intestines. Also, the anus might develop inflammatory signs from the irritation of the straining and from the elimination of hard pieces of stool.

Without treatment the animal will turn weak and lethargic, and vomiting may set in. The intestinal mucosal lining dehydrates, and the normally eliminated metabolic byproducts remain in the body. When they accumulate for too long, a type of self-poisoning occurs. This can lead to peritonitis and to death!

Causes
Most frequently constipation is caused by dietary mistakes, such as too much bone and too little fiber or too much dry food with too little water intake.

A lack of exercise may also be the cause. Running stimulates the digestion.

Other causes of constipation are painful anal conditions, overmedication, and disorders of the digestive secretory functions.

There are, also, mechanical causes, such as foreign bodies, intestinal occlusions, tumors, diverticulosis, paralysis, or perforations.

In the dachshund breed, specific paralysis may be accompanied by constipation. The same may occur in other breeds where orthopedic problems of the pelvic region create an unfavorable condition for the intestine.

Self-Help
Important: If your dog tends to have hard stools, do not feed it bones, raw meats, or organ meats.

If the food you have been feeding your dog contains rice, reduce the rice because it enhances constipation. Prepare the food more like a thick soup, and add some bran and thistle oil. You should also increase the dog's outdoor activities.

● Home Remedies
In order to reactivate the digestive processes, administer Nux vomica-Hcc drops, Rumisal drops, or Heelax-pills. For suggested dosages, see the inside front cover.

When to Consult a Veterinarian
Get help if the stool does not return to normal after one day, when the animal appears lethargic, or when a loss of appetite or vomiting becomes part of the symptoms. The latter may indicate an intestinal occlusion.

You also need to consult a professional if you are sure that the constipation is not caused by dietary factors, such as bones or too much dry food.

If in addition to constipation the animal shows signs of difficulties in getting up or walking, take your dog to a veterinarian trained in holistic techniques immediately.

What to Expect

Homeopathic single remedies will be employed to regulate the metabolic processes. Nosode therapy will be used to detoxify the body. If a bone or joint problem is present, acupuncture will be useful.

You will be asked to assist in the recovery process by learning how to administer color therapy and acupressure at home.

If the cause of the problem turns out to be a foreign body, you will be referred to a veterinary clinic for surgical removal of the object.

Preventive and Convalescent Care

If you know that your dog tends to have hard stools, you should eliminate bones from its diet.

Diseases of the Urinary Tract and Reproductive Organs

Urinary Incontinence

This term includes the uncontrolled release of urine ranging from dribbling to full bladder emptying.

Symptoms
While the animal is resting there is urine dribbling from the urethra. This may be the beginning phase of a chronic condition that acerbates and develops into chronic dribbles, and then into full voiding incidents.

Unless there is an inflammatory urinary tract condition, there should be no pain associated with incontinence.

Causes
In the aged dog incontinence may be caused by neurologic disorders that affect the muscle control in the bladder. Urinary tract inflammations are also frequently at the root of the problem.

Incontinence has also been observed following abdominal injuries, as well as a sequel to castration.

Self–Help
Important: Prevent your dog from resting on cold surfaces.

● **Home Remedies**
Give your dog one tablet of Cantharis D12 three times each day.

When to Consult a Veterinarian
After 14 days of unsuccessful home treatments you should take your dog to a veterinarian trained in holistic techniques.

What to Expect
Homeopathic single substance preparations will be put to work in order to regulate various organ functions. Toxins will be eliminated by the use of Nosode therapy. You will be asked to aid the treatment success by applying color therapy at home.

Preventive and Convalescent Care
Do not allow your dog to lie on cold surfaces.

Stay away from castration unless there is a medical reason for this procedure.

4

Inflammation of the Prepuce

While this condition is basically harmless, it turns into a nuisance for the pet owner because a discharge drips continuously from the dog's penis.

Symptoms
There is a continuous, creamy, yellowish discharge from the penis. In the beginning phase dripping is associated with movement. Later the discharge occurs even while the dog is lying down. The dog is found licking his penis continuously.

In some cases the discharge may be thick, green-yellow, and odorless, while in other cases it may appear liquid, odorous, and irritating to the skin. If the condition remains untreated in the early stages, it is likely to turn into a chronic problem that rarely responds to therapy.

Causes

Most preputial inflammations are caused by bacteria. Sometimes the inflammation may be caused by penile hairs that become retracted into the prepuce and cause irritations in their contact area. Lack of hygiene of the penile skin is another frequent cause that can be prevented.

Self-Help

Use diluted Calendula essence to rinse the space between the prepuce and the penis by squirting the liquid through a 10cc syringe. The dog must be lying on its side for this procedure. Place a flat container under the penis and squirt the solution gently into the tissue pocket between the penis and the prepuce. Hold the opening closed gently between your fingers, and massage the area carefully backwards. Then allow the liquid to empty into the catching container. The previously colorless liquid should now be milky or cloudy. In this way you are rinsing out the bacterial contamination. Repeat the procedure, and perform the treatment twice each day.

● **Home Remedies**

For internal treatment administer Pulsatilla-Injeel orally once each day for one week.

● **Bach Flowers**

Crab apple has proven to aid the healing process.

When to Consult a Veterinarian

If your home treatments have not yielded recovery after two weeks, you should consult a veterinarian trained in holistic techniques. Should the color of the discharge change to clear or show blood, you should take your dog to a veterinarian.

What to Expect

First, the affected organ will be thoroughly cleaned with specific antibacterial preparations in order to get rid of the infectious organisms. Then homeopathic remedies will be administered in order to enhance the body's own immune defenses and to fight the inflammatory process.

If an organic disorder is suspected, natural remedies will be employed to reestablish normal function, and Nosodes will be administered to enhance the elimination of toxins.

You will be asked to assist the recovery process by applying color therapy at home.

Preventive and Convalescent Care

After every walk or outing rinse your dog's penile area with a little tepid water. Trim any long penile hairs to prevent them from causing irritations. During moist spring and fall months limit the time your dog lies in grassy areas because there will be disease causing bacteria in the damp grass during these seasons.

Cystitis

Cystitis changes the pattern of urine elimination. Left untreated, this problem results in chronic bladder disease.

Symptoms

While the dog shows urges to urinate there are only a few drops being released. The color of the urine may be milky or yellowish and may be mixed with blood. Pain is frequently obvious during elimination. Other symptoms may accompany this disease, such as fever, weakness, lack of appetite, or vomiting.

Causes

The main cause of cystitis is the combination of cold and wet weather, and a habit of lying on cold surfaces. While the dog rolls around in wet grass or on other soiled surfaces it is easy for the penile area to pick up a host of bacteria that may enter the urinary tract through the urethra. Dogs who are often prevented from relieving themselves in a timely manner may incur muscular retention disorders that, in the long run, cause cystitis.

Self-Help

Important: Quiet rest in a warm location is the number one requirement for dogs with cystitis.

● Home Remedies

Spascupreel tablets are indicated for dogs who show signs of painful spasms during urination. If there is evidence of light red blood in the urine, prepare a mixture of Berberis D12 and Cantharis D12 drops. Suggested dosages are on the inside front cover.

Twice a week you should administer Solidago comp. orally in order to prevent an advancing kidney infection.

● Bach Flowers

Hornbeam and olive are recommended if your dog appears listless due to the cystitis.

When to Consult a Veterinarian

Make an appointment when the cystitis has not improved after two days of treatment, or if the general condition of the dog gets worse.

What to Expect

Homeopathic single remedies will be employed to strengthen the general condition and to rid the body of the infection. In addition, Nosode therapy will stimulate the elimination of toxins. You will be able to aid recovery by applying color therapy.

Preventive and Convalescent Care

Try to prevent your dog from exposure to cold and wet surroundings.

Taking your dog for regular and frequent walks will enable the animal to empty the bladder fully.

Kidney Diseases

There are three basic types of kidney disorders that you might encounter in your dog: inflammation, degeneration processes, and stone formations. Kidney disorders are relatively common in dogs.

Symptoms

(A) Nephritis is an inflammatory disorder of the kidneys. It is characterized by fever, weakness, increased thirst, and equally increased urination, as well as by moist eczema, hair loss, and ear inflammation. The latter is usually located on the left side. The dog's coat appears dull, and the white of the eyes turns red. After a short while inappetence may set in, and the animal may start walking with an arched back and a stiff gait. If you exert pressure in the area of the kidneys, the dog will respond with pain. Sometimes vomiting and diarrhea may accompany the syndrome. The dark colored urine may be tinged with blood. Later in the course of the disease, urination will decrease, which leads to a buildup of toxins in the body and to uremia.

(B) Degenerative disorders of the kidneys (nephrosis) are marked by a combination of weight loss with the formation of an enlarged belly (ascites). The animal will drink a lot of water, the urine will appear milky, and as the disease progresses, the mouth of the dog may have a urinelike odor.

Important: Take your dog to a veterinarian trained in holistic techniques immediately if the described symptoms occur.

4

(C) Male dogs are more often affected by kidney stones (nephrolithiasis) than females. This condition is painful during urination. The flow of urine may stop or slow to a dribble, and it may contain blood.

Causes

Kidney disorders are caused mostly by an accumulation of toxins in the body. This occurs as a reaction to an underlying disease like tonsillitis, a cold, or an abscessed tooth. If a dog suffers from cystitis, there is a chance that bacteria from the bladder has ascended to the kidneys causing nephritis.

The kidneys can also be damaged by the following causes: spicy foods, too much dry kibbles, canned foods without sufficient water consumption, food that is too rich in fats or proteins, or foods that are too high in chemical preservatives.

Malfunctioning of the parathyroid glands can also lead to kidney disorders.

Self-Help

Feed your dog a diet that is low in proteins (see page 106). Supervise the intake of plenty of fresh clean water. Take your dog for as many walks each day as possible so there is ample opportunity for the dog to void all of the urine. Any retention may be harmful at this time.

Important: A warm and quiet place to rest is now of utmost importance.

● **Home Remedies**

Reneel tablets will assist the general improvement of kidney function. Use Spascupreel tablets if painful cramping is evident. For blood stained urine, Cantharis D12 tablets are indicated. You can improve the kidney's cellular functions and condition with a biweekly dose of Solidago comp. orally. For suggested dosages see the inside front cover.

● **Bach Flowers**

Hornbeam or olive will strengthen a weak and lethargic animal, and crab apple will aid the internal cleansing process.

When to Consult a Veterinarian

When the symptoms outlined in (B) above are observed you should take your dog to a veterinarian trained in holistic techniques immediately. The same is true for cases where the general condition of the animal is not noticeably improved after five days of home treatments or if vomiting and fever accompany the other symptoms.

What to Expect

Homeopathic single remedies will be selected for the regulation of urine production and elimination. For detoxification the specialist will employ Nosode therapy.

If nephrosis is suspected, cytoplasm therapy will be administered in order to stimulate regenerative processes in the kidney. To aid the recovery process you will be instructed in the application of color therapy.

Preventive and Convalescent Care

Prevent your dog from lying on cold or wet surfaces, and make sure that the animal has access to plenty of fresh drinking water.

Increased Sexual Drive

Increased sexual orientation toward the other gender occurs mainly in male dogs. This condition is considered mostly an inherited trait.

Symptoms

The affected animal frequently whines and urges the owner to let it go outside. Once outside the dog seeks the scent of a female, whether she is in heat or not. If a female is accessible, the dog will try to mount her at all cost.

Another expression of the problem is for the dog to get into the habit of licking his penile area continually, which frequently leads to painful irritations and inflammations. Eventually the dog might refuse food. If the condition affects a female dog, the animal usually expresses it by trying to mount any human leg that walks in her way.

Causes
Most conditions of this type are hereditary.

Self-Help
● **Home Remedies**
There is no remedy for an increased sexual drive. The focus must be placed on the regulation of hormone function and production.

For female dogs administer Hormeel drops two to three times each day. Male dogs should receive Platinum C 200 drops once each week.

If continued licking has caused additional inflammation of the penis or prepuce, apply a cleansing rinse with Calendula essence (see self-help for Inflammation of the Prepuce, page 62).

● **Bach Flowers**
Mustard will lift the spirits of a depressed patient, while vine is indicated for the more tyrannical one.

When to Consult a Veterinarian
Get professional advice if your home treatments do not control the excessive sexual behavior of your pet.

What to Expect
High potentiated homeopathic remedies will be employed to lower the sexual response pattern.

Preventive and Convalescent Care
If you have the time, play with your dog and offer as much distraction as possible.

If you have a female dog in heat, it would be best to curb exposures to males as much as possible.

A dog who tries to mount human legs should be discouraged by consistent correction that teaches the animal not to exercise this behavior!

The Heat Cycle

A dog is in heat when her estrous cycle prepares her to accept males for mating. The first heat usually occurs between the sixth and the eleventh month of age. The subsequent heat cycles can be expected twice each year. The heat cycle lasts about 21 days. The dog stands for males mostly from the ninth to the fifteenth day after the onset of estrus, which frequently coincides with evidence of bleeding. During this time you must guard your dog carefully if you want to prevent a pregnancy.

During a normal heat cycle the dog's vulva appears swollen and warm, which gave the scientific term "estrus" its lay term "heat." First secretions are mostly dark red in color, but they change to pale red and finally are colorless after the eighth day. A white mucoid discharge is often more scent attractive to males than the early red secretions.

Normal heat cycles can induce variable appetite patterns, as well as a lack of discipline. While she will "stand" for the male to mount her when the critical stage of the cycle is reached, she will fight off any male when the time is not right for mating.

Symptoms
(A) Irregular heat cyles: The dog is in heat more often or less often than every 6 months; or the dog bleeds too much or too little (silent heat).

This type of hormonal imbalances are particularly annoying if you plan to breed your bitch.

(B) Pseudopregnancy: Your dog's behavior changes about eight to ten weeks after she was in heat. If she had mated this would be the time she would give birth. Despite the fact that she did not mate she is now beginning to build a nest, she hides, and whines, and holds on to her toys in her basket. She appears overly affectionate. In addition the mammary glands may become enlarged, and may even produce small amounts of milk. This condition may last from two to four weeks. A serious inflammation of the mammary glands (mastitis) can develop if the bitch starts to suck on her own teats. Fever, listlessness, and inappetence might accompany the list of symptoms. In the worst case the uterus could become involved in the inflammatory disease (pyometra).

Causes

Both disorders, irregular estrus, as well as pseudopregnancy, are caused by functional disorders of the hypophysis, the uterus, or the ovaries.

Self-Help

If your dog suffers a pseudopregnancy, you should distract her as much as possible, and keep her away from all her toys until the condition has passed. If the mammary glands are swollen and hot, you should make cool compresses soaked in alcohol or Calendula essence.

You may try to have your dog volunteer as a foster mother for somebody's orphaned pups. During the duration of the pseudopregnancy the diet should be low in rice and pasta. Your dog should not drink too much during this time. Do not add milk to the diet.

Important: Do not squeeze the nipples to check for milk flow, and prevent the animal from licking or sucking her own nipples. You need to prevent the development of a mastitis.

● **Home Remedies**

(A) Use Hormeel drops to regulate the hormonal balance.

(B) If your pet turned into an overaffectionate lover, treat her with oral administrations of Pulsatilla ampules. If she becomes overly reserved, give her Sepia ampules orally. For suggested dosages see the inside front cover.

Important: Should you notice an acute change in your dog's general well-being, such as inappetence, depression, or vaginal discharge, you should treat her first, and immediately thereafter take her to a veterinarian trained in holistic techniques. As a treatment you should administer oral ampules of Pyrogenium-Injeel and Lachesis-Injeel, twice each day. A veterinarian must be consulted to determine whether uterine disease is the problem.

● **Bach Flowers**

The suggested Bach flowers are indicated for pseudopregnancy and irregular estrus cyles.

If the dog acts	Administer
Overly affectionate	Centaury, cerato, or heather
Resentful, offended	Pine
Dominant, aggressive, proud	Beech, chicory, and water violet

When to Consult a Veterinarian

If a Hormeel treatment is not effective and if general symptoms appear in conjunction with the pseudopregnancy, call a veterinarian trained in holistic techniques.

What to Expect

Homeopathic single substance formulations will be chosen specifically to treat the hormone imbalance and generally for overall strengthening. You will be instructed in the use of color therapy in order to aid the recovery process at home.

Weak Labor Contractions

Uterine contractions are the beginning of the birthing process.

Symptoms

Contractions might be underway for several hours, yet no pup has emerged. This is usually a sign of an acute problem. The cause may be uterine inertia, i.e., insufficiently strong contractions to expel the pup. You may find your bitch in an exceedingly weak condition.

Causes

Most cases of uterine inertia are caused by hormonal disorders.

Self-Help

Important: The suggested medications are to be used only for the immediate emergency situation until you have reached a healthcare professional. These remedies are not adequate as treatments.

● Home Remedies

Caulophyllum C30 and Secale-cornutum C30 should be given every thirty minutes. Change from one to the other remedy every half hour. This medication will restimulate the labor contractions.

● Bach Flowers

If your pet is very weak, give her hornbeam and olive. After the pups are delivered give her walnut.

When to Consult a Veterinarian

Get help immediately from a veterinarian trained in holistic techniques.

What to Expect

Homeopathic single remedies will be selected to remove the birthing obstacles. If the medications are not effective, the bitch will be prepared for a cesarian section by a veterinarian.

Preventive and Convalescent Care

If you are dealing with an animal that has had previous birthing problems, it would be advisable that you have a professional check the animal from time to time during the pregnancy.

Lactation

Symptoms

(A) If the bitch does not produce enough milk, she cannot feed her litter.

(B) If there are too few pups to drink all of the produced milk, there will be an excess.

Causes

(A) Lack of milk production is most commonly due to hormonal imbalance. In some cases it can be caused by poor nutrition during pregnancy.

4

(B) In most cases there are not enough pups to drink all of the existing milk. One or more pups might have died.

Self-Help
If you cannot find a foster mother for your pups, you need to feed them with mother replacement milk. This product is comercially available in pet stores.

● Home Remedies
The bitch should be treated with a single dose of either one tablet or five to ten drops of Urtica-urens C30.

● Bach Flowers
Revive your weak and exhausted animal with hornbeam, olive, and walnut.
(B) If your bitch has too much milk, offer her as a foster mom to orphan pups. If this does not work out, give her Urtica-urens D6 three times each day for a few days.

When to Consult a Veterinarian
Get help from a veterinarian trained in holistic techniques if your home remedies are ineffective.

What to Expect
Homeopathic single remedies will be employed to strengthen the overall condition of the animal, as well as to rebalance the hormonal system. You will be instructed in the use of color therapy and in the application of acupressure.

Preventive and Convalescent Care
Place the whelping box in a room where the mother can take care of her pups without worrying about disturbances.

Mastitis

This problem predominantly affects those bitches that tend to have pseudopregnancies.

Symptoms
The mammary glands are swollen and hot. They may feel soft or hard, and they may be red. The nipples may show secretions that could contain pus. This inflammatory condition renders the animal weak and listless.

Causes
Mastitis is commonly caused by either an infection, an impact, or pressure.

Self-Help
Place cool compresses, soaked in Calendula or alcohol, on the affected mammary glands, and give your dog absolute bed rest.

Important: Prevent your patient from licking the affected areas. This will aggravate the inflammation.

● Home Remedies
Administer one tablet of Traumeel three times per day. If the condition is very painful, add oral doses of Bryonia-Injeel, and if the swelling is soft and not sensitive, add Apis-Injeel orally.

● Bach Flowers
Hornbeam is indicated if the dog is tired and listless.

When to Consult a Veterinarian
Get help immediately if a fever develops.

What to Expect

Homeopathic single remedies will be administered in order to treat the inflammation, to stimulate the body's own defense mechanism, and to correct any hormonal imbalances.

You will learn how to apply color therapy to aid the recovery process.

Prostate Disease

Mainly older male dogs suffer from an enlarged and/or inflamed prostate.

Symptoms

An enlarged prostate condition is usually recognized by your dog's changed behavior. The tail is kept abnormally high, and the gait is very halting and stiff. Your first thought will be that the animal is suffering from a musculoskeletal disorder. The next sign is a pencil-thin stool formation, which is caused by the pressure of the prostate on the intestine. Elimination is difficult or not successful at all. In some cases there are additional symptoms, such as a bloody or suppurative discharge, or blood tinged urine. While prostate enlargement is commonly painless, there is a chance it will develop into prostate inflammation (prostatitis), which happens frequently in males with increased sexual drive.

Inflammatory prostate disease is very painful. It is accompanied by fever, thirst, lack of appetite, and vomiting. The animal has great difficulties in getting up, or lying down. Climbing stairs and walking or jumping become almost impossible.

Important: If the condition remains untreated, accumulation of inflammatory toxins might lead to polyarthritis.

Causes

Prostate disease is generally age related. Only very rarely is this disease caused by a bacterial infection.

Self-Help

Important: The suggested remedies are indicated for prostate enlargement only. For prostatitis disease you need help from a health professional.

Give your dog increased outdoor activities in order to empty the bladder and to prevent internal pressure. Prepare a diet that is easily digestible, and do not feed bones. This will ease defecation.

● Home Remedies

Administer five to ten drops of Prostagutt three times daily. If the improvement is not pronounced after 14 days, change to Nettisabal drops using the same dosage.

● Bach Flowers

Hornbeam and mustard will enliven a tired animal and if the dog is hyperactive, treat him with vervain. An impatient patient should be treated with impatiens.

When to Consult a Veterinarian

Get help if you suspect prostatitis. The same is necessary if your remedies have not improved the condition of the prostate enlargement.

What to Expect

Homeopathic single remedies will treat the inflammation, while Nosode therapy will eliminate the accumulated toxins. In addition, there are homeopathic cell substances available that can be employed to improve the damaged prostate cells, and cytoplasm therapy is effective in stimulating regenerative processes.

4

You will be instructed in the use of color therapy.

Preventive and Convalescent Care
Keep up a consistent schedule of daily short walks and specific diets.

Diseases of the Testicles

Disorders of the testicles include inflammatory diseases, tumors, and eczema.

(A) Testicles appear enlarged and painful. The animal is hesitant when getting up. It will walk stiffly and with the legs as far away from the painful testicle as possible. This gait is the cause of frequent misdiagnosed cases because the dog is thought to have a back problem or some type of hindleg paralysis.

Important: If the condition is caused by a testicular tumor there are commonly other symptoms in addition to the above: hair loss, enlarged nipples and/or an enlarged abdomen. This disease affects mainly older male dogs. Take your animal to a specialist as soon as you notice these symptoms.

(B) The dog continues to lick his scrotum because the skin itches. The licking causes a moist eczema. You need to stop the licking habit in order to prevent bleeding and pus formation.

Causes
(A) Inflammatory testicular disease may be a sequel to injuries or to general infectious diseases, such as brucellosis or tuberculosis.

(B) Scrotal itching is most commonly caused by increased sexual drive.

Self-Help
(A) Prepare cool compresses soaked in Calendula or Hamamelis dilutions. Then rub the affected scrotum gently with Traumeel ointment or with Rescue cream.

Important: You must prevent the dog from chewing or licking its testicles.

● **Home Remedies**
(A) Administer Traumeel tablets if the testicles appear hot to the touch, reddened, or swollen. In addition, treat the dog orally with Calcium iodatum-Injeel and with Conium-Injeel.

(B) Administer daily drops of Cosmochema Skin Function, which will improve the skin functions. Add Croton D12 tablets to the treatment. For suggested dosages, see the inside front cover.

● **Bach Flowers**
If your dog appears listless and lethargic due to its health problem, treat it with hornbeam and olive.

When to Consult a Veterinarian
Homeopathic single remedies will be selected to treat the acute condition of the disorder. This is followed by the use of Nosode therapy in order to detoxify the body. Finally, you will be instructed in the use of color therapy to continue home treatments.

Preventive and Convalescent Care
The dog must be prevented from chewing or licking his testicles. Occupying him in a variety of ways will distract him.

Diseases of the Skin and Glands

Dander (Seborrhea)

Dander is most frequently associated with metabolic disorders.

Symptoms
The skin produces dander either in particular parts of the body or all over. The back and pelvic areas are usually more affected than other areas. Dander may appear fine and dry on dry skin, or it may feel greasy on equally greasy skin. Itching may be associated with dander, and an intense "dog odor" is typical for this problem.

Causes
Wrong foods often cause dander, or it may appear as an allergic reaction to something.

Other causes are disorders of the liver functions, or hormone and glandular disorders.

Dogs that are exclusively kept indoors may end up with dry, flaky skin without actually being sick.

Self-Help
If you have been feeding a uniformly repetitive diet, change it by adding some variety.

Important: Whenever you change the diet, do so slowly, over some time in order to prevent diarrhea.

● Home Remedies
Administer Cosmochema Skin Function drops or Psorinoheel to support a balanced metabolism. Suggested dosages are on the inside front cover. To treat dry dander, use 5–10 drops of Dermisal daily. If the skin is greasy, give your dog an oral ampule of Arsenicum album-Injeel every day.

When to Consult a Veterinarian
Get help if the condition persists beyond two weeks despite your treatments, and if the animal appears generally sick.

Depending on the severity of the dog's condition, you may need to consult a veterinarian sooner than two weeks.

What to Expect
A veterinarian trained in holistic techniques will select specific homeopathic single remedies to regulate metabolic functions, and Nosode therapy will be employed to detoxify the body. You will be taught how to use color therapy at home in order to speed the recovery process.

Preventive and Convalescent Care
There is no better preventive care than a correct diet (see page 14) and a maintenance schedule (see page 104) that best fits your particular dog.

Sufficient outdoor activities are important to stimulate a healthy metabolism.

5

Warts

Warts are benign hypertrophic elevations of the top skin layers. They may appear all over the body, and they are most frequently found in old dogs. They do not affect the general health of your pet.

Symptoms

At first you will notice only a little bump in the skin. The bump can get quite large, and it can turn into a soft skin appendage, or it may form a hard wart while others end up shaped like a cauliflower.

Causes

Warts are either inherited or they can be the result of age related weakened tissue conditions.

Self-Help

As topical treatment you should dab the warts with a lightly diluted tincture of Thuja.

Important: Do not try to remove the warts because you will risk causing an inflammation!

● **Home Remedies**

The remedy is selected according to the type of warts.

Type of Wart	Oral Treatment
Soft meaty warts	Dulcamara-Injeel
Hard stem appendage	Causticum-Injeel
Cauliflower shaped warts	Thuja-Injeel

Dosages are on the inside front cover

● **Bach Flowers**

Give crab apple to aid the treatment.

When to Consult a Veterinarian

Consult a veterinarian trained in holistic techniques if the warts continue to grow despite your treatments, or if the warts begin to change color and shape.

What to Expect

Through the use of high potentiated homeopathic single remedies the general organism of the dog will be strengthened, which will prevent further growth of the warts.

Allergies

Most allergies are inherited but some may be activated by exposure to certain irritants.

It is wise to examine your dog regularly and keep a record or your observations.

Symptoms

Itching is usually the first sign of an allergy. Moist or dry eczema follow, as well as swelling and reddening.

Other typical signs are watery eyes, a runny nose, coughing, vomiting, or diarrhea.

If the dog is reacting to a medicine or to overmedication, the animal's head may swell up. This looks like the dog's head is enlarged, and you will notice thick folds on the forehead.

Causes

The animal could react to a variety of agents: environmental agents, such as pollen or dust; medications; food components like wheat, milk, or the ingredients of commercial dry or canned food; and, last but not least, insect stings.

Self-Help

You should feed your dog a special diet (see page 106).

Important: Avoid food that contains poultry and veal because these meats could increase the itching.

● Home Remedies

Oral administration of Engystol ampules will induce an unspecific detoxification process in the body. Pro-Aller drops will regulate a variety of metabolic disorders, and Cosmochema Skin Function drops are very effective in diminishing the itching problem.

To treat a localized swelling or irritation like an insect sting, you can orally administer ampules of Apis-Injeel.

Thuja D30 is indicated for a reaction to a medication.

Frubiase-Calcium ampules are highly effective for all sorts of allergic reactions. Suggested dosages are on the inside front cover.

● Bach Flowers

Whatever the cause, give your dog crab apple. Hornbeam will lift the spirit of a listless patient, and cherry plum is indicated for a dog that is getting highly agitated because of bad scratching fits.

When to Consult a Veterinarian

If the allergic reaction continues beyond two or three days, a veterinarian specialist should be contacted to establish the origin of the problem. Get help immediately if the general condition of the animal worsens.

What to Expect

Homeopathic remedies will strengthen the overall condition of the dog while the use of Nosode therapy will eliminate toxins from the body. In some cases the use of desensitization injections may be indicated (see page 120). This treatment is not available everywhere.

Preventive and Convalescent Care

If your dog tends to have allergic reactions, you should, above all, make sure that the diet contains as little chemical preservatives as possible. A good balanced diet is the top requirement (see page 14).

Breed Dispositions

German shepherds, poodles, boxers, and dalmatians tend to have more allergies than other breeds.

Hair Loss and Hair Damage

Dogs normally change their coat twice each year, in the spring and in the fall. This is a normal physiological process. Sometimes the hair loss may be excessive, or it may be accompanied by other symptoms. Hair loss that occurs outside of the normal time pattern is usually caused by metabolic disorders.

Symptoms

(A) The dog loses hair excessively throughout the year.

(B) The dog loses hair evenly, all over its body. The brush is full of hair after every combing session, and the skin appears dry and flaky. In some cases the animal has lost much of its appetite, and constipation, as well as general malaise, may be part of the picture.

(C) There is a sudden onset of hair loss accompanied by itching, eczema, dander, and a dulling coat. Broken hair may occur chronically. In the latter case the hair grows just above the skin and then it breaks off.

(D) Hair loss occurs in specific limited areas of the body, and these areas itch. Upon closer inspection there is evidence of reddish brown dots, black particles, or small bumps in the skin.

5

(E) Hair loss occurs evenly all over the body. The dog scratches and develops eczema. Sometimes diarrhea will occur.

(F) Bare spots develop under the collar, the muzzle, or the harness. Itching, skin irritations, and sometimes diarrhea are part of the syndrome.

(G) When you pet your dog you end up with a whole bunch of hair in your hand. While a health care specialist examines your dog, hair falls out in bunches.

Important: Dogs with symptoms (B) and (E) must be treated immediately. If it is left untreated, the animal will develop serious secondary infections because the skin is lacking its normal acid balanced protective coating.

Causes

(A) This is usually a problem that occurs in dogs that are kept indoors most of the time.

(B) This pattern is mostly due to a diet consisting exclusively of canned or kibbled food.

(C) These cases are predominantly caused by liver disorders, or by incorrect diet. If kidney disorders are causing the hair loss, there will be evidence of moist eczema. Hormonal causes will show the hair loss at the inside of the thighs and around the genitalia. Hormonal imbalance of the thyroid or the hypophysis will lead to hair loss symmetrically on both sides of the vertebral column.

(D) The dog is infested with ectoparasites (see page 79).

(E) Bacteria or fungi are the probable causes.

(F) The respective accessories are too tight or too rough. The hair loss is caused by pressure and rubbing.

(G) Shock and stress can lead to sudden acute hair loss.

Self-Help

Important: Dogs with symptoms listed in categories (C) and (E) above should be presented to a veterinarian trained in holistic techniques immediately for diagnosis of the cause of the problem.

(A) Take the dog for extensive walks in order to stimulate the metabolic activities of the skin. Regular brushing also enhances the blood circulation of the skin, and at the same time it removes dead hair. Treat your dog by adding Biotin to the food.

● **Home Remedies**
Use Cosmochema Skin Function drops, and add Sulfur-Injeel in case of dander.

● **Bach Flowers**
Administer crab apple to support internal cleansing.

(B) Your dog is showing a reaction to certain additives in commercial food. Begin to change the food slowly toward fresh meats, vegetables, rice, and low fat cottage cheese.

(D) Formulation-Z tablets will change the scent on the surface of the skin, which the parasites can't stand. Find the parasites in the coat (see page 81). Use diluted Calendula essence for topical treatment of the affected areas, and follow up with a thin coat of Rescue cream.

(E) To aid the detoxification process give your dog Toxex drops.

(F) Remove the mechanical irritation by loosening the accessories or by replacing them. Dab the irritated and inflamed areas with Calendula essence and follow up with a thin coat of Traumeel ointment.

(G) If you know that your dog is reacting to stress or trauma, administer Rescue drops (Bach flowers). Suggested dosages are on the inside front cover.

When to Consult a Veterinarian

Seek the professional help of a veterinarian trained in holistic techniques if your home treatment is unsuccessful within one week, if the condition is getting worse, or if eczema or other symptoms develop.

What to Expect

Homeopathic single remedies will be employed to strengthen the dog and to reestablish a balanced hormonal system. If toxins are the causes of the hair loss, the veterinarian will apply Nosode therapy to cleanse the body.

Preventive and Convalescent Care

Consistent care of the coat combined with a correct diet (see page 14) are the best preventive measures you can take.

Breed Dispositions

German shepherds and chow chows tend to be more affected by hair loss than other breeds.

Eczema

Eczema is an inflammatory condition of the skin that develops pus if it is not treated. A lowered immune system condition will encourage formation of eczema. Eczema can also be an expression of the body's reaction to toxins.

Symptoms

There are two types of eczema. One type is moist, contains pus, and can be foul smelling. The other type is dry and flaky.

Important: You must be aware of the location of the eczema. If it occurs symmetrically it is important for the veterinarian to know because it will affect the choice of treatment.

Eczema usually itches and causes the dog to scratch, lick, and chew the affected areas excessively. This spreads the condition even further. Bacterial infections will follow causing pus or pustules to form in small or extended areas. Depending on the type of infection, the color and consistency may range from white to greenish pustules, to yellow or brown creamy pus. You should try to keep a record of your observations.

Causes

Metabolic disorders are the most common causes of eczema formation.

Frequently, the disorder begins with an incorrect diet, which leads to liver and kidney disorders. When the body can no longer manage the elimination of toxins, the skin will try to take on that task.

Moist, suppurative eczema indicates kidney disorders, while dry, flaky eczema commonly follows liver function problems.

Other common causes are bathing ponds that are heavily contaminated, and the disposition of dog breeds that have heavily folded skin that invites bacterial growth.

Hormonal imbalance causes symmetrical eczema in conjunction with hair loss.

Parasites can also cause eczema (see pages 56, 79).

Self-Help

Important: Do not treat eczema with a layer of ointments! You will make the condition worse. These lesions need air to heal.

While your dog suffers from eczema it is best to remove meats from the diet and to increase rice, vegetables, and low fat cottage cheese. If you must feed meat to your dog, use lamb. If diet was the problem in the first place, make the transition to a proper diet slowly.

Treat the eczematous skin areas daily with diluted Calendula essence. If the lesions are moist, spray them with Dr. Schaette Wound Balm before you take the dog outdoors. This will prevent secondary bacterial infections.

● Home Remedies

In addition to the topical treatment you should provide your dog with a systemic detoxification therapy. You should begin with Toxex drops.

After five days you will need to change to a medication that is specific for the type of eczema your dog has. If the skin lesion is moist, you should administer Psorinoheel drops. If it is a dry eczema, use either Dermisal drops or Sulfur-Injeel ampules.

In all cases of skin disorders you can use Cosmochema Skin Function drops.

If you are dealing with an advanced suppurative eczema, Staphylosal drops or Hepar sulfuris-injeel are indicated.

Suggested dosages are on the inside front cover.

● Bach Flowers

Crab apple is most useful to strengthen the overall condition of the animal.

When to Consult a Veterinarian

Get help if the animal shows general symptoms of illness in addition to the skin condition.

What to Expect

Pathogens that are responsible for pus formation need to be eliminated by Nosode therapy. In addition, homeopathic single remedies will stimu-late the body to use its own immune system to fight the infection.

If major organ disorders are at the root of the problem, the application of cytoplasm therapy will encourage regenerative functions in the affected organs. It might be necessary for you to use color therapy, so you can assist the recovery process at home.

Preventive and Convalescent Care

A balanced breed specific diet is the best prevention of disease.

Pay special attention to hygiene in your dog's environment! You should routinely examine your pet for any skin abnormalities.

Breed Dispositions

The skin folds of some dog breeds make them more susceptible to moist eczema than other dogs.

Abscesses

There are acute inflammatory abscesses that are warm to the touch and chronic abscesses that are cold to the touch.

It is important to examine your dog regularly for any skin abnormalities.

Symptoms

The affected area is red, swollen, warm, and painful. If you try to touch the area, the animal may bite as a reaction to the pain.

If you suspect that your pet is in pain, take great care when examining it. You may also want to ask someone to assist you.

If the infection is carried over into the general organism of the dog, it may experience fever, weakness, inappetence, or even blood poisoning.

Causes

Abscesses are usually caused by a local injury that allows bacteria to enter the lesion as it would happen in a bite wound. An acute abscess can develop into a chronic lesion.

Self-Help

If the abscess is not fully developed, Calendula compresses will help the progress, or you can bandage the abscessation with Traumeel ointment.

If you are dealing with a mature abscess, you should place compresses with Luvos Heilerde (mud) on the affected area, and, after you take the compress off, cover it with a thin layer of Ichtholan ointment.

● Home Remedies

At first treat your dog with Hepar sulfuris-Injeel or with Staphylosal drops. If the swelling has not subsided after two days, or if the abscess is not fully mature after one week, change the medication to Myristica-sebifera D12 tablets. Once the acute inflammation is finished, Silicea-Injeel, or Traumeel tablets will help the final healing process. Suggested dosages are on the inside front cover.

● Bach Flowers

If your patient is grumpy or moody because of the pain, lift its spirits with willow. Impatiens are helpful for the irritable and impatient animal.

When to Consult a Veterinarian?

Get help from a professional if the general condition of the animal changes, if the inflammation does not recede after treatment, or if the abscess does not mature within one week.

What to Expect

Homeopathic single remedies will fight the inflammation, and Nosodes will eliminate toxins from the body. To aid the healing process you will be instructed in the use of color therapy.

Chewing Paws

When dogs chew their paws they injure the skin and cause serious inflammations due to the bacteria that settle in the wounds.

Symptoms

Despite the lack of any obvious external reason the dog chews
(A) on all paws.
(B) on either hind or front legs.
Inflammation only occurs after protracted repetitive injury.
(C) and nibbles conspicuously between the toes. Upon inspection there are small red dots and red areas visible. The same type of dots are found on the belly and on the inside of the thighs. The dog might have been lying on a lawn.
(D) or licks a specific area of one paw. That area is red and swollen.

Causes

(A) This may be an important sign that the animal feels neglected and bored, and it is trying to get attention.
(B) Metabolic disorders are at work here. The hind paws are usually affected if the kidney is dysfunctional, and the front paws are the victims of liver disorders.
(C) Grass mites are commonly the culprits of the small red dots (see page 79).
(D) This type of chewing most commonly follows an injury by either a foreign body, a tear or cut,

5

or by an insect sting. If the lesion is open, it is probably infected by bacteria.

Self-Help

Dab the affected areas of the paws or beteen the toes with diluted Calendula essence, and let it dry. Don't let the dog lick the fluid off otherwise you lose the effect. The essence is not harmful though! If you can clearly see the inflammation, cover the sore area with Dr. Schaette Wound Balm before every outdoor activity.

In addition to this topical treatment, there are special measures you can take for each type of lesion.

If your dog is bored, you need to provide distraction and occupation.

If your pet feels neglected, you might need to change your relationship and interactive behavior.

You can try behavioral training if all your other efforts fail to help the dog.

● Bach Flowers

Crab apple is good in any case for internal cleansing.

If the dog appears to be	Administer
Lacking willpower	Centaury
Insecure	Cerato
Craving attention	Chicory
Overaffectionate	Heather
Jealous	Holly
Impatient	Impatiens
Inferior to other animals	Larch
Hopeless	Sweet chestnut
Hyperactive	Vervain
"A little tyrant"	Vine

If the condition is due to a metabolic disorder, use Hepar-comp. ampules if the front paws are affected and Solidago comp. ampules if the hind paws are affected to assist renal metabolism. Either medication should be given orally, at the rate of $^1/_2$–1 ampule three times each week.

Important: If you suspect a metabolic disorder and you have been feeding mainly commercial diets, this is the time to introduce a slow change to fresh foods!

(C) If your dog gets infested with grass mites frequently, you need to initiate a change in the overall metabolic patterns. Start the treatment with five Psorinoheel drops three times each day. If this does not show results within one week, you need to change to giving one Sulfu-Injeel ampule orally every other day.

(D) Traumeel tablets (one tablet 3–5 times daily) are most effective in case of injuries, pain, and irritation. After you clean the affected area with Calendula essence you can cover it with a thin layer of Traumeel ointment, or you can use Rescue cream.

Important: Do not bandage the lesion after you cover it with a thin film of ointment!

When to Consult a Veterinarian

Get professional help if all four paws are affected. The cause is probably a serious metabolic disorder. Also make an appointment if your treatments have not yielded success or the initial inflammations turn into pus.

What to Expect

Classic homeopathic remedies will be selected to treat potentially underlying metabolic disorders and to ameliorate inflammatory processes. The use of Nosodes will affect the elimination of toxins that might be introduced by bacterial infections. If metabolic disorders are diagnosed, the specialist will instruct you in the application of acupressure.

Preventive and Convalescent Care

Prevent your dog from licking and chewing in order to avoid serious infections.

Wrong nutrition may have led to metabolic disorders. If you think that this might have been the case, begin a slow change to a high quality diet. There is no better disease prevention than a good diet (see page 14).

After each outing wash your dog's paws with warm water, and dry them thoroughly. Treat your dog like a living creature—not like an object!

Parasites (Ectoparasites)

Just about all dogs get in contact with ectoparasites during their lives. This does not pose a problem to a healthy dog!

If, however, your pet is repeatedly affected by parasites, it is likely that it has an impaired immune system.

Important: Parasites transmit diseases! Fleas transmit the dog tapeworm, and ticks transmit Lyme disease. The latter is a serious illness marked by recurring fevers.

Symptoms

The dog scratches either in one particular area or all over the body. Scratching leads to inflammation and to itching eczematous reactions (see page 75), often accompanied by loss of hair (see page 73).

Recurring parasitic infestation may lead to vomiting, fever, and exhaustion, even to convulsing episodes. The latter symptoms are often mistaken for other disease symptoms.

Severe metabolic disorders may develop after prolonged parasitic infestation.

Causes

The most common ectoparasites in a dog's coat are *fleas, lice, ticks*, and *mites*.

Fleas are easily seen running and jumping on the dog's body and in the dog's sleeping quarters. They also leave their tracks by depositing their excrements in the form of tiny black clumps that cling to the hairs of the dog.

Lice can also be seen easily. They accumulate preferentially around the neck and above the upper lip. They crack when you squeeze them between two fingernails. Their eggs are attached to the coat.

Ticks attach themselves by burrowing their head in the dog's skin. They suck blood until they have increased their size by several times, and then they fall off. They usually leave behind a small nodular skin reaction. Ticks are concentrated mostly along the neck and head of the dog. Certain ticks are particularly dangerous in that they may carry Lyme disease.

Mites are tiny and hardly visible (*grass mites*), or not visible at all (*mange mites*).

Grass mites appear mainly in the spring when you can recognize them around the mouth and between the toes of your dog. They look like little red dots. They are also attracted to the inner thigh and to the belly. The genital areas may also be affected.

There are mainly two mange mites that affect dogs, the *Demodex* and the *Sarcoptes* mites. Demodex invades the hair follicles causing dandruff, hair loss, and secondary infections with pus formation. The Sarcoptes mites dig into the top skin layers and deposit their eggs. The resulting itch becomes an almost unbearable irritation for the dog. These mites most frequently affect the front paws, ears, eyes, and the root of the tail.

5

Important: Sarcoptes mites are transmissible to humans, where they cause severe itching rashes. If you suspect mange mites on your pet you should consult a veterinarian trained in holistic techniques immediately.

Self-Help

Formula-Z tablets have proven to be highly effective as a natural tick prevention (see page 8). Should you still run into a tick on your dog's body, remove it with a tick forceps. If the head is not fully extracted, it can lead to a bad inflammation.

Tick collars make no sense at all because their chemicals will be absorbed through the skin. Some dogs also react allergically with itching and hair loss.

There are, unfortunately, no herbal cures for lice, fleas, and mites. However, the preventive effectiveness of Formula-Z tablets (see page 8) appears to be quite favorable in the experience of many practitioners.

If your dog requires a chemical treatment for severe infestation, you will need to aid the detoxification process. This will protect the dog from incurring secondary diseases. Give your dog for one week, once, every other day, 5–10 drops of Sulfur C30, or you can give Dermisal instead. Discontinue the treatment slowly over several days.

● **Bach Flowers**
Administer crab apple to support psychological well-being.

What To Expect

Most probably the specialist will apply Nosode therapy for the elimination of toxins. Homeopathic remedies will be selected that will regulate metabolic imbalances. You will be instructed in the use of color therapy.

Preventive and Convalescent Care

During the spring season and any other time when parasites are prevailing, mix Formula-Z tablets into your dog's food as a preventive measure. Even if there are no ticks around, the tablets won't harm your pet.

Look for signs of parasites when you brush your dog and inspect his coat and skin on a regularly basis. This is particularly important if you live in an area with many bushes, trees, and grassy areas.

Try to avoid letting your dog go for a run in wooded areas—especially if Lyme disease is a problem in your area.

Inflammation of the Anal Sacs

The anal sacs are located on either side of the anus. They empty normally while the dog eliminates. In some dogs the impaired function of these sacs leads to an inflammatory condition because the secretions are retained.

Symptoms

The most typical picture for this condition is a dog that is trying to slide along the floor on its hindquarters (see sledding, page 110).

In addition, the dog bites and licks the anal surroundings continually or in sudden spurts. It looks like the dog is chasing its tail, while in reality, it is trying to deal with the irritating itch of the inflammation.

The animal has obvious discomfort during elimination, as well as expressing pain as a reaction to any touch in that area. The anal sac area emits a very repugnant smell.

If the anal sacs are occluded, the condition will develop into a fistula, severe inflammation, and pus formation.

Causes

During episodes of diarrhea and while a dog eliminates mainly soft stools, there is a lack of pressure stimulation that normally induces the anal sacs to empty. Hereditary dysfunction may cause a similar problem.

Self-Help

Cleanse the anal area with diluted Calendula essence and follow up carefully placing a thin coat of Hamamelis ointment on the anus.

It is also a good idea to keep the hair around the anal area short to prevent matting and caking with fecal matter and anal sac secretions.

● Home Remedies

Give your dog one tablet each of Traumeel and Paeonia three times each day. If the animal is very sensitive to touch, add one ampule of Hepar sulfuris-Injeel each day.

When to Consult a Veterinarian

Get help if your treatments are ineffective after five days.

What to Expect

If the anal sacs are occluded, the veterinarian trained in holistic techniques will express and irrigate them. The veterinarian will use homeopathic single remedies to treat the pain and to lower the inflammation. You may then be asked to support the therapy by administering color therapy at home.

Diabetes Insipidus

This disease causes a loss of fluid regulation in the body. It is referred to as diabetes insipidus, and it affects mainly old dogs.

Symptoms

All at once the animal starts to drink as much as several liters of water. It urinates proportionally as much. The urine is clear and watery, and the dog needs to go outside even during the night.

A typical symptom that accompanies this disease is a dull, dry, and rough coat.

The tissues are drying out, especially the mouth.

As the condition progresses, the animal becomes listless, loses weight, and has a lack of coordination.

Blindness will possibly also occur.

Causes

Diabetes insipidus is, as a rule, caused by a disorder of the hypophysis. At the root of the problem may be a cancer or an adrenal tumor.

Self-Help

Important: Home remedies are not suitable in these cases. The help of a veterinarian is advised.

● Bach Flowers

Olive and hornbeam are helpful to enliven a tired and listless patient.

When to Consult a Veterinarian

Get help as soon as you notice that the animal drinks an extraordinary amount of water.

What to Expect

Homeopathic single remedies will be employed to regulate the hypophysis and the adrenal glands. For the improvement of damaged cell functions the use of homeopathic cell products and cytoplasm therapy will be considered.

5

Breed Dispositions

Poodles and boxers carry hereditary dispositions to this disease.

Diabetes Mellitus

Diabetes mellitus is a disease that is caused by a lack of the hormone insulin. Insulin is manufactured in the pancreas. Diabetes is diagnosed mainly in older dogs.

Symptoms

Increased thirst and frequent urination are hallmarks of this disorder.

Also typical is a fruity odor from the mouth of the dog, and the coat will appear dull.

Despite a healthy appetite, the animal will lose weight.

As the disease progresses, other symptoms will occur, such as overall itching, vomiting, apathy, and accelerated breathing.

Corneal clouding and eventual blindness may also develop.

Excessive fluid loss may cause a dog to succumb to a coma and death. It is therefore important to keep track of your dog's bodily functions.

Causes

This disease is caused by a lack of insulin production by the pancreas. It is either congenital or it develops due to malfunctioning of the pituitary gland.

Other potential causes are: wrong diets, pregnancy, pseudopregnancy, stress, and reactions to chemical substances.

Self-Help

The dog needs a protein-rich diet unless kidney problems exist simultaneously.

Important: Feed the dog small meals several times each day. This won't be a problem if your dog is used to eating at a specific time each day. If, however, you have let your dog have access to his food at all times and he is now at an advanced age, it may take some time to regulate his food. Your veterinarian may be able to give you some advice in this area.

● **Home Remedies**

Syzygium comp. drops have proven highly effective at a dose of 5–10 drops, 1–3 times each day.

When to Consult a Veterinarian

As soon as you notice any signs of diabetes take your dog for a professional evaluation of the stage and background of the disease.

What to Expect

Homeopathic single remedies will be employed to restimulate the pancreas while homeopathic cell preparations will be administered to rebuild the organ structure.

You will be asked to assist the therapy progress by applying color therapy at home.

Depending on the severity of the disease, you may be asked to administer daily insulin injections to your pet.

Preventive and Convalescent Care

You should provide a top quality diet and prevent obesity.

Breed Dispositions

Diabetes occurs more often in dachshunds and spaniels than in other breeds.

Neurologic and Orthopedic Diseases

Muscle Ache

Symptoms
The dog shows some difficulties in getting up and hesitates to start moving. This occurs mostly on the day following a lot of exercise.

The same symptoms appear when the animal suffers from arthritic disease (see page 84). The difference lies in the duration of the conditions. The muscle ache is acute and diminishes soon while the arthritic problem persists.

Causes
Muscular exertion causes muscles to ache by accumulating metabolic acids in the tissues.

Self–Help
Important: Do not overexercise your dog now, but do not allow the animal to lie still altogether. Take the dog for several short walks rather than for one extended outing. Short light exercise will regulate the muscle metabolism.

● Home Remedies
You can aid the muscle tissue by administering one tablet of Arnica C30 each day.

Preventive and Convalescent Care
Be careful not to overexercise a dog that is not used to it. Increase exercise slowly.

Disc Prolapse

This problem mainly affects dogs with very elongated backs. It is a very painful condition that leads to hindleg paralysis if left to develop into a chronic ailment.

Symptoms
The beginning phase is highly painful with a sudden onset of paralytic episodes. Stair climbing becomes very difficult, and the animal begs to be carried.

When you pet the animal along the back you will notice that the musculature contracts like in a spasm.

As the dog tries to walk the hindlegs seem to slip away from under the body.

With progressive disease the animal can no longer move the hindlegs due to paralysis. It moves by pulling itself forward with front legs, sliding the lifeless hind quarters behind the body. In these late stages all sensitivity and reflexes have vanished.

At this time the animal has lost control of urination and defecation. Urine and stools may either flow uncontrolled or may be retained due to a lack of muscle innervation.

Causes
Progressive paralysis is caused by a disc prolapse, which is due to wear and tear of the vertebral column. This condition worsens with age. However, a sudden abrupt and forceful motion can cause the same injury.

6

Self-Help

Important: Absolute rest is indicated only in the beginning phase. Later, you need to take the animal for many short and slow walks in order to prevent the degenerative loss of muscle tissue. Any extra body weight should be reduced in order to relieve stress on the skeletal system.

● Home Remedies

Treat the dog with Colocynthis-Hcc drops, and orally add Discus-comp. ampules twice each week. In cases where the animal has difficulties with elimination, use Nux vomica-Hcc drops. During the painful beginning phase treat the dog with Traumeel tablets, and orally with Hypericum-Injeel ampules. For suggested dosages see the inside front cover.

● Bach Flowers

Bach flowers will help you with the improvement of the animal's psychological condition.

If the dog appears to be	Administer
Listless, uninterested	Hornbeam
Easily panicked	Rock Rose
Impatient	Impatiens
Hyperactive	Vervain
Moody	Scleranthus

When to Consult a Veterinarian

Get help as soon as your dog shows signs of impaired mobility or paralysis.

What to Expect

Cytoplasm therapy will be used to stimulate the regenerative processes in the vertebral column. Laser acupuncture will be employed to unblock the vertebral meridians, and homeopathic single remedies will be administered to relieve the pain and to strengthen the overall conditions of the animal.

To complement the treatments vitamin B supplements will be prescribed, and you will be instructed in the use of color therapy, as well as acupressure techniques for home treatments.

Preventive and Convalescent Care

If you own a dog of the predisposed breeds, you should make it a rule not to teach your pet tricks that involve "sitting up," or jumping onto any furniture.

Stair climbing should be kept to a minimum.

Watch your pet's food intake to prevent it from gaining extra weight.

Breed Dispositions

Disc prolapse is a problem that mainly affects dachshund and other chondrodystrophic breeds (see page 120), such as Pekingese, French bulldogs, basset hounds, spaniels, beagles, and poodles.

Arthritis

The symptoms of arthritis and arthrosis look alike, but only arthritis is an inflammatory disease.

Symptoms

The joints appear swollen and warmer than normal. Sometimes the animal runs a fever. If the condition is an arthrosis the dog has no problem getting up and moving around. After a while of walking, however, the animal begins to limp.

In many cases there is only one joint affected, while in others many joints are affected simultaneously *(polyarthritis)*.

Causes

Arthritis is most often preceded by a generalized inflammatory disease that sends out toxins into all of the joints. An injury can also lead to an inflamed joint. The latter must be remembered even if a long time has passed between the injury and the appearance of arthritic symptoms.

Self-Help

Take your dog for short walks to allow it some exercise but prevent any unnecessary stress on the joints.

Important: Your pet needs alot of rest now! Reduce the meat content in the diet, and increase the vegetables, rice, and low fat cottage cheese.

● **Home Remedies**

Give your dog one Traumeel tablet three to five times each day, one to two Zeel tablets three times each day, and one Bryonia-Injeel ampule each day.

● **Bach Flowers**

If the animal reacts with depression to the arthritis, give it hornbeam and olive.

When to Consult a Veterinarian

Get help if your treatments do not lead to improvement.

What to Expect

Homeopathic single remedies will positively stimulate the overall functions of the body. Nosode therapy will detoxify the organism, and with cytoplasm therapy the joints will be stimulated to regenerate. You will be advised how to use color therapy and acupressure in order to aid the recovery process.

Preventive and Convalescent Care

Prevent your dog from overexertions.

Arthrosis

Arthrosis refers to joint conditions that are caused by wear and tear and that are mostly associated with aging. While a cure is not available, home remedies help to alleviate pain and discomfort.

Symptoms

There is clear evidence that the animal feels discomfort in getting up and during the initial moments of moving about. The dog appears stiff and limps at first, then, slowly straightening out, the animal walks normally. After an extended walk, pain sets in, and the animals starts limping again. Cold and damp weather commonly aggravate the problem.

Causes

This condition is caused by wear and tear. The fluid that is normally produced in the joints (synovia) is being used up too quickly. This is an age related problem, but it can be caused in young animals by overextending their joint activities. In some breeds this condition is hereditary.

Self-Help

Important: Keep your walks short and do them more often. They should be no longer than ten to twenty minutes at any time.

Mix a bag of gelatin into the food. To fortify the connective tissue give your dog ATR20 or ATR9 with the food. The dosage should be according to body weight.

6

● Home Remedies

Use one to two Zeel tablets three times each day. In addition, give your dog one to two Traumeel tablets several times a day. To help further you can add a daily tablet of Rhustoxicodendron C30.

● Bach Flowers

If your pet appears unresponsive, encourage it with hornbeam. Use mustard, if it looks sad or depressed. Willow is indicated when your dog is in a bad mood.

When to Consult a Veterinarian

If your treatments remain unsuccessful, and if the condition gets worse, get professional help. Also do so if the legs seem to sink away uncontrollably from under your dog.

What to Expect

With the aid of classical homeopathic remedies the overall condition, as well as general mobility, will be improved.

Laser acupuncture will be used to unblock meridians along the joints, and to enhance this treatment you will be instructed in acupressure techniques.

In addition, cytoplasm therapy will be employed in order to improve the quality and attachment of the joint-associated cartilage, muscles, and tendons. This treatment will alleviate the discomfort.

Color therapy should also be part of the treatment.

Preventive and Convalescent Care

If you know that you have a dog with an inherited disposition, make it a rule from the beginning that the animal will not be overexercised or encouraged to jump.

You should provide a firm mattress for your dog to prevent it from lying on cold surfaces. You should prevent overweight conditions, and if the animal is already overweight, you should reduce dietary calories.

Dogs with congenital arthrosis should not be allowed to reproduce!

Breed Dispositions

Arthrosis affects mainly large and heavy breeds that suffer predominantly from hip dysplasia. Old age arthrosis, however, may affect all types of dogs.

Neuralgia

Neuralgia refers to painful conditions that are not necessarily associated with movement, but which may attack the animal without warning.

Symptoms

The animal is heard vocalizing suddenly, and it avoids any movement at this moment.

Sometimes the pain will cause it to snap at anyone who tries to touch it.

Causes

The pain results from an inflammation of nerves. Drafts could be one of the causes. However, toxins somewhere in the body may also lead to nerve inflammation.

Important: If left untreated, neuralgia may lead to serious nerve disorders, including paralysis.

Self-Help

Important: The animal must have total rest!

● Home Remedies

Give your dog one tablet of Hypericum D4 several times each day. If the pain seems to extend into the neck and head areas, add Gelsemium-Hcc drops to the treatment. If, however, the pain appears to be localized more towards the back and pelvic areas, use Colocynthis-Hcc drops. Suggested dosages are on the inside front cover.

● **Bach Flowers**
Hornbeam will lift the spirits of a listless and depressed patient.

When to Consult a Veterinarian
Get help if your remedies are not effective within four to five days.

What to Expect
With the help of homeopathic single remedies the overall condition of the animal will be strengthened, and Nosode therapy will be employed to eliminate the toxic burden.

Laser acupuncture will unblock the affected nerve meridians. You will be instructed in the use of color therapy and acupressure so you can aid the recovery process.

Preventive and Convalescent Care
Prevent your animal from exposure to drafts and to cold and damp conditions.

Breed Dispositions
Shorthaired breeds are disposed to neuralgia.

Convulsions, Cramps

Spasms or cramps and convulsions refer to muscle contractions of variable intensity involving all of the body. Dogs of all ages may be affected.

Symptoms
(A) Convulsions run through the whole body. In addition, you will notice a blank stare and pale mucosals.
(B) The dog has repeated convulsions. In the beginning, each attack lasts only seconds, or, at the most, one minute. Left untreated, the intervals between attacks become shorter with time, and the episodes last longer.

In most cases the animal acts slightly nervous prior to an attack. In the midst of perfect well-being, the animal suddenly halts, stares blankly ahead, and the pupils widen. Subsequently the animal collapses, stretching its limbs with spastic rigidity. Muscle contractions, head torsion, and foaming salivation follow the collapse. The animal may void urine and stool. It is unconscious. The animal might accidentally bite its tongue during the convulsion, which would cause the saliva to be mixed with blood.

After an attack the animal behaves normally, and does not appear to remember anything. Hunger and thirst are commonly increased after an episode. Because each attack is responsible for the loss of a certain number of brain cells, it is possible that the animal may develop behavioral changes as the condition progresses.
(C) The dog crouches and whimpers indicating pain in the abdominal area. In most cases the condition passes as soon as the dog moves or if a stool is passed.
(D) There is evidence of muscle contraction in the area of certain joints.
(E) Convulsions occur following a vaccination.

Causes
(A) This condition is caused by either injuries or tumors of the brain or by a lack of oxygen access to the brain. Other causes are infectious diseases like Leptospirosis, Aujeszky disease, or

6

rabies, as well as poisoning, metabolic disorders, or severe worm infestation.

(B) This picture is almost exclusively seen in epilepsy. This is a congenital disease. There are some cases where epileptic types of convulsions are seen following bacterial infections by flea or tick bites. The latter must be distinguished from a true epileptic attack by a veterinarian.

(C) Bloating and intestinal cramps are usually caused by wrong foods or by endoparasites.

(D) Mineral deficiency is the cause in this case.

(E) This symptom is caused by an adverse reaction to the vaccine.

Self–Help

Important: Do not try home remedies for cases with symptoms shown in (A). Treat your dog with Rescue drops and get professional help.

(B) If at all possible, move your dog to a dark room during an attack. Position the animal in a way that it cannot injure itself. Talk to it calmingly, stroking it reassuringly. Administer Rescue drops as soon as the animal regains conscious-ness. Every 15 minutes place one pulverized tablet of Belladonna D12 on your patient's tongue (see page 102). This occasion does not lend itself to the administration of drops because they contain alcohol. After each attack add ½ ampule Cerebrum-comp. to the treatment. This will protect the brain tissue.

(C) During the first two hours administer one Spascupreel tablet every 15 minutes. During the following days, while the symptoms persist, give the dog three tablets each day. Then, slowly taper off the medication until it is stopped.

(D) Administer one Magnesium-Verla pill one to two times each day. Calm the animal, and lightly massage its limbs stroking towards the heart.

(E) Administer a single dose of one Thuja-Injeel ampule.

● **Bach Flowers**
In all cases cited above, it has proven helpful to add Bach flowers to the treatment. Each condition requires the choice of specific Bach flowers.

When to Consult a Veterinarian
In cases listed under (A) get help right away. All of the other conditions should also be seen by a veterinarian trained in holistic techniques.

What to Expect
With the use of Bioresonance analysis the origin of the problem will be established. Classic homeo-pathic single remedies will strengthen the overall condition of the body in order to increase the intervals between convulsions. Cytoplasm therapy will protect and improve brain cell functions.

If there is evidence of toxins in the body, the veterinarian will use Nosode therapy to eliminate them. You will be asked to assist the recovery through color therapy.

Preventive and Convalescent Care
(A) Formula-Z tablets protect the dog against ticks. Do not forget the required rabies booster vaccination!

(B) Avoid any kind of stress and excitement to prevent the onset of an attack.

(C) and (D) A high quality diet is the best prevention (see page 14).

Breed Dispositions
Golden retrievers, poodles, schnauzers, and dachshund tend to be more affected than other breeds.

Psychological Illnesses

Fear

Your dog depends on your help to overcome fear! The psychological stress of continued fear can harm the organic health of your dog.

Symptoms

(A) Your dog hides, trembling, maybe whimpering in a corner, each time there is a strange or loud noise. It is difficult to convince the animal to come out of hiding.

(B) Whether they are people or other dogs, your pet is frightened by them each time.
Your dog reacts with fearful demeanor every time it is taken to an unfamiliar environment.

(C) The dog barks threateningly at every other dog "Don't get any closer to me!" Even very small dogs bark like this at large strangers.

(D) When you walk your dog it is likely to be aggressive toward humans and animals alike.

Causes

(A) Some dogs are born fearful.

(B) The dog was exposed to a psychological trauma or to a frightening experience at an earlier age in its life. Such trauma can block normal behavior. Any new environment scares the animal.

(C) "Fear biting" is an aggressive expression of fear. The normal expression would be flight.

(D) The dog's protective behavior on your behalf is strongly expressed toward others.

Self-Help

Important: Never chide a fearful animal! No matter how minor the incident might seem to you, the animal would lose its trust in you.

● **Home Remedies**

If your dog is nervous and fearful-hyperactive, try a treatment with Nervoheel tablets. This will gently calm the internal unrest.

● **Bach Flowers**

The dog	Treat the dog with
Specific fear	Mimulus and Rescue drops
General fear	Aspen and Rescue drops
Posttraumatic fear	Star of Bethlehem
Indecision	Cerato
Feeling of inferiority	Larch
Overprotectiveness	Red chestnut
Panic	Rock rose
Overexcitement	Cherry plum

Rescue drops are indicated only in cases of emergency. They should be stopped as soon as the behavior has normalized.

When to Consult a Veterinarian

Prepare for an office call if your dog has not shown any improvement within four weeks of home treatment.

7

What to Expect

High-potentiated homeopathic medications are indicated to regulate psychological imbalances. You may be asked to aid the treatments by using color therapy at home.

The veterinarian trained in holistic techniques will help you in the selection of Bach Flowers for your dog's specific needs.

Preventive and Convalescent Care

Above all, you need to inspire trust between youself and your four-legged friend. If you are not quite sure what exactly will be in the best interest of your dog, you might consider attending a dog training course.

Breed Dispositions

Miniature breeds show a relatively high incident of congenital fearful behaviors. Pet owners have to pay close attention to their interactions with their dogs. Mistakes could harm the psychological well-being of a sensitive animal.

Jealousy

Dogs may react with jealousy to changes in your personal world.

Symptoms

(A) The dog becomes aggressive. The dog growls and tries to interfere with the person whom the animal considers an intruder. It will do anything to defend the way things were before when its place in the hirarchy was not challenged.

(B) The dog persists in drawing attention to itself by asking to play, by being overaffectionate, or, finally, by beginning to chew on itself.

(C) The dog starts to behave obstinately, and it might defecate or urinate inside the house, despite the fact that it has always been house-broken.

(D) The dog acts offended. It refuses food and hides in a corner.

Causes

All of the above cited symptoms have the same cause. The dog is jealous because it has to share your affection or attention. This could be caused by a friend, a baby, a spouse, or even by an object.

Self-Help

Give your pet as much attention as you did before the change occurred, and find ways to reassure the animal that it has retained your love.

Talk to your dog as much as you can. This will give the animal a feeling of being included, and it will adapt more easily to the new situation.

● Bach Flowers

Bach Flowers are uniquely suited for the purpose of balancing a disturbed psyche.

Symptoms	Treatment
(A)	Holly
(B)	Heather
(C)	Vine, crab apple
(D)	Mustard

Remember to use consistency in your training efforts.

When to Consult a Veterinarian

Make an appointment if your dog's behavior has not responded to Bach flowers within three weeks.

Homesickness

Symptoms

(A) The animal whines, becomes aggressive, or tears up toys or other objects.

(B) The dog retreats and appears depressed. It refuses food and is unresponsive to enticements.

(C) The normally housebroken animal defecates or urinates inside the house. If this behavior continues without treatment, the dog may become so sick psychologically that it will mutilate itself by chewing through its skin and creating serious self-injury.

Causes

The most common cause for homesickness in young dogs is the separation anxiety caused by weaning and relocation away from its family pack.

In adult dogs homesickness occurs most frequently when their master is away from home for a prolonged absence. Some dogs do not adjust well to their temporary homes, be that a friend's house, a dog motel, or your relative's apartment.

Self-Help

● **Home Remedies**

Administer Ignatia ampules orally.

For suggested dosages see the inside front cover.

● **Bach Flowers**

Use Rescue drops if the puppy is being separated from its mother. If the dog is aggressive, give it holly, and if your pet appears sad, mustard and hornbeam are indicated. Obstinate behavior should be treated with vine, and if the dog is craving attention, treat it with heather.

When to Consult a Veterinarian

If the animal continues to refuse food and becomes more unhappy, you need to get professional advice in order to avoid the development of serious organic disorders.

What to Expect

Homeopathic remedies will be selected that will restabilize a psychological imbalance.

Preventive and Convalescent Care

Before you leave for a prolonged absence it would be best if you could get your dog well-familiarized with its temporary caretakers and environment. This will create the necessary trust and reassurance.

If your problem child is a new puppy, you should spend as much time together as possible, especially during the first week. Only close contact and reassurance will help the little fellow over its painful separation.

Neutering or Sterilizing

If you do not want to breed your dog there are several options.

(1) You can try to keep your female away from encounters with males twice each year for the 10 or more days while she is in heat.

(2) You can have the female spayed.

(3) You can have a male dog castrated.

(4) If the dog has been mated unintentionally, you can have her treated with a hormone injection to prevent pregnancy. This is not a good solution except for emergencies because it enhances your dog's susceptibility to cancer and diabetes.

If (1) is excluded, you should get the animal sterilized, castrated, or spayed. Sterilization involves the severance of the oviduct of a female and the severance of the vas deference in the male. Castration is referred to as the removal of the testicles in the male. Spaying, or ovariohysterect-

7

omy, refers to the removal of the ovaries and uterus in the female.

Neutering may result in behavioral changes such as lethargy or lazy and listless attitudes. Urinary incontinence may also be observed (see page 61). The altered hormonal system may in some cases lead to skin disorders. Homeopathic and other home remedies are not indicated because the organs that would need to be stimulated are removed. In order to replace the missing hormones they must be injected.

If your dog underwent a neutering procedure (whatever the reason) and you observe the symptoms described above, seek the advice of a veterinarian as soon as you can. Homeopathic single remedies may be selected that will attempt (!) to stimulate the remaining hormonal systems (e.g., the adrenals) to participate in the production of sex hormones. In order to revitalize a potential weakness of the hypophysis, the veterinarian trained in holistic techniques can apply the use of homeopathic cell preparations, and, to stimulate regenerative processes, cytoplasm therapy might be used.

Surgeries

For the treatment of some diseases nothing can prevent the use of anesthesia and/or surgery. A tooth extraction or the removal of tartar would fall into this group.

Even if your dog undergoes surgery or an anesthetic procedure in a veterinary clinic, you can aid your patient's recovery by administering home remedies.

Treating your dog before the surgery will enable the animal to tolerate the anesthetic procedure much better, and the psychological stress is greatly reduced.

Home treatments after the surgery will minimize the anesthetic effects, and it will greatly aid in the recovery and healing processes.

Presurgical Care
Approximately thirty minutes before the anesthesia is scheduled you can administer five drops of Rescue (Bach flowers) medication. Dilute the drops in one teaspoon of bottled spring water, and place the liquid inside the mouth. Add 5–10 drops or one tablet of Arnica C30.

Warning: Check with a veterinarian first. Any physical alterations prior to anesthesia could alter the actions of the anesthetic agents used and pose an anesthetic risk. It depends on which agents are to be used.

Postsurgical Care
As soon as your animal arrives back at home, repeat the administration of Rescue drops and Arnica. Susequently, continue treatment for three days with one tablet of Traumeel five times each day. On the following three days give one Traumeel tablet three times each day. After that, slowly taper off the treatment until you can stop altogether.

Aid in Dying

Advanced age, serious disease, or accidents may hasten the end of a dog's life. During this final phase of your friend's life it is most important that you give the animal all the possible comforts and affection. When you recognize that there is no recovery possible, it would appear to be misled love to allow your pet to suffer a slow death. You may ask a veterinarian to come to your house to put your dog to sleep with a euthanasia injection. A house call would spare your beloved friend the stress of being taken to a strange environment.

Before euthanasia is to be performed, you may want to give your dog Rescue drops. This Bach flower treatment has a calming effect on an animal that instinctively knows that "something is going to happen." The drops will help to make the experience gentle and peaceful.

In chronically ill animal patients and in old dogs it is very difficult to arrive at a timely decision as to when euthanasia is the appropriate end to suffering. If you recognize that the animal's will to live has diminished, it is time to say good-bye. A pet owner can tell this stage because the dog no longer responds to invitations to play. Bach flowers make the passage gentle and smooth. If you are not sure about your dog's will to live, you can test this also with Bach flowers. Administer a single (!) dose of two drops each of olive, hornbeam, walnut, and wild rose mixed with one tablespoon of water. If your dog remains lethargic or unresponsive thirty minutes after the treatment, there is not enough strength left in the animal to make it feel better. In this case you should proceed with the application of the following formulation. Add five drops each of walnut, Rescue, and aspen to 10 ml of plain water. Do not use alcohol. Give your dog ten drops of this mixture every thirty minutes. While some dogs fall asleep peacefully after the second dose, other animals need a varying number of administrations.

In many cases the veterinary injection will no longer be needed because the Bach flowers may instead help the animal "bounce back."

Bach flowers do not kill the animal. They do, however, help in the process of letting go.

7

Emergencies

Internal Bleeding

Internal bleeding may originate in the ears, nose, mouth, or intestines. Such incidents must be immediately presented to a veterinarian.

First Aid

Administer immediate first aid by giving your dog, 3, 5, or 10 drops of Rescue drops, depending on its size.

Stop a nose bleed by pushing a small vinegar soaked cotton ball into the bleeding side of the nose.

External Bleeding

Causes of external bleeding episodes: cuts, bites, stabs, scrapes, scratches, and eczema.

First Aid

Carefully cut the hair around the bleeding area. Then clean the skin by dabbing it with diluted Calendula essence and let it dry.

If the injury is small, just spray a little Dr. Schaette Wound Balm on the affected tissue. This will disinfect the wound.

For a large wound, place a sterile compress on it and secure it with a gauze bandage, winding it crosswise in the direction of the heart.

● Home Remedies

If you are dealing with a bite wound, give your dog one tablet of Traumeel every fifteen minutes.

● Bach Flowers

Depending on your dog's size, administer 3, 5, or 10 drops of Rescue drops and of crab apple.

Burn Injuries

First Aid

Apply cold water or ice immediately. Wrap ice cubes in a wash cloth.

● Home Remedies

Depending on the dog's size, administer 3, 5, or 10 drops of Causticum comp., as well as 0.5 ml Echinacea comp., four times daily (use one ampule).

● Bach Flowers

Depending on the dog's size, administer 3, 5, or 10 drops of crab apple to support your dog's overall condition.

If the burn caused deep tissue damage, apply a sterile compress to cover the injury and take your dog immediately to a veterinarian.

Heatstroke/Sunstroke

Typical symptoms are: sudden fainting, collapsing, rapid pulse rate, fever, and/or very pale or bluish white mucosal surfaces.

First Aid

Remove the dog as quickly as possible to a shaded or cool, dark area. Place cool wet cloths on its body. Take the animal as soon as it is practical to a veterinarian.

● Home Remedies

Administer an emergency treatment consisting of one tablet Apis C 30 and one ampule of Aconitum-Injeel.

● Bach Flowers

If the dog is deeply lethargic, instill a mixture of wild rose, hornbeam, and olive. To alleviate the emotional trauma, use star of Bethlehem at a dose of 3, 5, or 10 drops depending on the size of the dog.

Poisoning

General symptoms are salivation, foaming at the mouth, vomiting, or blood in the vomit or urine.

First Aid

Induce vomiting by administering approximately 50 ml of saltwater (one teaspoon of salt per 50 ml of tepid water). Inject this through a syringe into the mouth (see page 102).

● Home Remedies

Administer a single dose of Nux-vomica. Use any dilution you happen to have available. In addition, give your dog one tablet of Okoubaka D4 every five minutes.

For poisoning caused by ingestion of spoiled meats, treat your pet with Arsenicum album-Injeel ampules for drinking. Rat poison should be counteracted with Lachesis D30 tablets. Suggested dosages are on the inside front cover.

At all costs, you should take your dog to a veterinarian! If you know the causative agent, make sure that you take it along with you.

Insect Stings

First Aid

Cool the affected area immediately with ice. Keep the dog quiet and still to prevent the poison from being circulated in the body. If the sting is located in the neck or throat areas, cool the inside by allowing iced water to run slowly into the mouth while applying ice packs to the outside.

● Home Remedies

Administer Apis C30 in a singular dose of five to ten drops or one tablet.

● Bach Flowers

Treat first with Rescue drops, then follow up with a mixture of crab apple, star of Bethlehem, and wild rose. Use 3, 5, or 10 drops as needed.

Take the dog to a veterinarian immediately if lethargy, cramps, or vomiting occur.

8

Shortness of Breath

Symptoms: The dog is found on its side, rigid, and gasping for air.

First Aid

Carefully inspect the throat of the dog for a foreign object that might be lodged there. Remove any such findings. If you do not find an object, rush the dog to a veterinarian as quickly as you can.

● **Home Remedies**

Orally administer one ampule of carbo-vegetabilis-Injeel.

● **Bach Flowers**

To alleviate panic reaction that is caused by the inability to breathe, administer 3, 5, 10 Rescue drops as needed.

Paralysis

Causes for paralytic episodes range from impacts and accidents to toxins and infectious diseases.

First Aid

Immediate attention by a veterinarian is required.

● **Home Remedies**

In order to bridge the time period between home and clinic, you should orally administer one ampule of Hypericum-Injeel and one tablet of Arnica C30. If the paralysis is restricted to the front legs, treat the dog with Gelsemium-Hcc drops, while you would use Colocynthis-Hcc drops for hind leg paralysis. Use 3, 5, or 10 drops as needed.

● **Bach Flowers**

Olive and wild rose are indicated for signs of lethargy or unresponsiveness while rock rose is helpful in cases of panic. The dose ranges are 3, 5, or 10 drops depending on the size of the dog.

Loss of Consciousness, Fainting

First Aid

Call your veterinarian immediately.

Check the vital signs of your dog meticulously:

● *Breathing:* If the chest shows no signs of breathing, you must apply resuscitation measures. Place the dog on its side; hold the dog's lips and mouth shut while blowing forcefully for three seconds into the nasal openings; repeat this procedure several times until the chest begins to move, and you can see the dog breathing. After one minute, check whether the dog is breathing on its own; if not, continue your resuscitation efforts until the expert arrives.

● *If there is no mobile animal health care provider in your neighborhood, place the animal in a blanket and rush it to an emergency clinic.*

● *Heart Attack:* Place your hand flat on the left side of the chest. Feel the heartbeat and measure the heartbeats per minute (see page 97). Carefully examine the mouth and nose and remove any evidence of vomiting or other excretions that could block the airways. Pull the tongue gently forward and out to the side.

In order to stabilize the circulatory functions, immediately administer the contents of one ampule of carbo-vegetabilis-Injeel by dripping it between the lips. If you do not have this product, you can also use 3, 5, or 10 drops of Veratum-Hcc.

If you have to transport an unconscious dog, use a blanket as a stretcher. If you suspect a fracture of the vertebral column, place the dog on a wooden board for transport.

Measuring the Pulse

You can feel the pulse most easily in the middle of the inside thigh (see page 101). Place your fingertips gently on that area, until you feel the pulse.

Normal pulse rates range between 70 and 100 beats per minute. Large dogs have slower pulse rates than small dogs.

A pulse rate that is faster than 120 beats per minute is considered abnormal, and so is a rate slower than 60 beats per minute. It is a good idea to measure your dog's normal pulse rate when the animal is in good health, so that you will be able to recognize any abnormalities when they occur.

8

Practical Advice for Dog Owners

When we talk about diseases, we mean that certain organic processes are not functioning properly or that one or more organs are so badly affected that general physical and/or psychological changes occur. As a responsible pet owner, you should provide the quality of care necessary to prevent illness from developing. If your dog gets sick despite your best efforts, you will need to know how to act and what to do to speed the healing process. The following pages will guide you with advice and additional tips.

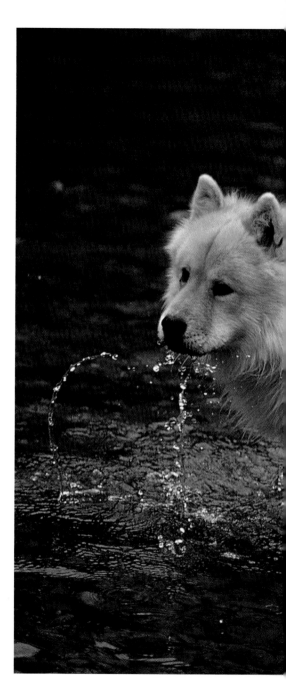

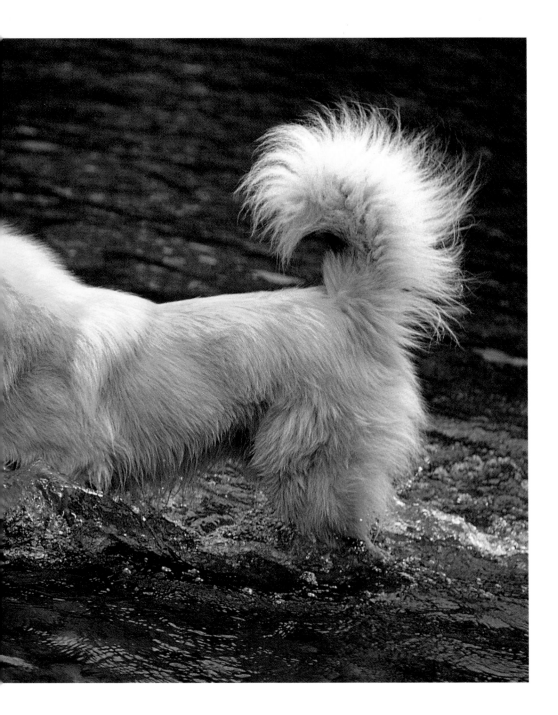

Practical Advice

First Aid

Any changes that you observe in your dog's behavior may be indications for a beginning stage of illness. It is important that you write down your observations because, at a later date, each notation may be valuable information for a veterinarian who is presented with the sick dog.

Measuring a dog's temperature and taking its pulse are two primary first aid procedures that you should learn and practice. They are essential to check a dog's general condition and to find out whether an illness is about to develop.

Taking the Temperature

Your best choice of thermometers is a digital model that sounds a signal when the temperature is fully recorded. Avoid the old fashioned thermometers which carry the risk of breaking and spilling alcohol or mercury, which is a poisonous substance. Broken glass adds another potential source of injury for the dog.

Switch the digital thermometer on, dip the point of the thermometer in a little petroleum jelly and insert it about one inch (2 cm) through the anus into the rectum. The petroleum jelly will prevent the thermometer from hurting the dog by sticking to the rectal mucosal lining. Once the signal sounds, retract the thermometer and read the temperature.

The normal temperature of a dog ranges from 100 to 102.5°F (38.6 to 38.8°C). Some small and exotic breeds may have temperatures as low as 99.5°F (38.2°C).

A dog is considered to have elevated temperatures beginning at 103°F (39°C). Any higher temperatures are considered fever and require treatment. An elevated temperature is usually an indication of a generalized inflammatory process in the body.

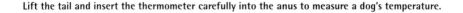

Lift the tail and insert the thermometer carefully into the anus to measure a dog's temperature.

Nature's Pharmacy

The best way to prepare for any emergencies is a well-stocked doggie medicine cabinet. Here is a list of nature's remedies that you should have on hand.

Products	Treatment of:
Apis C30 tablets	Insect stings
Calendula Tincture for external use	Cleaning and wound cleaning
Carbo-vegetablis-Injeel	Circulatory problems
Dysentery drops	Diarrhea
Euphrasia eyedrops	Eye irritations
Febrisal drops	Fever from 103°F (39°C)
Keratisal drops	Eye irritations
Okoubaka D4 tablets	Poisoning
Rescue drops	Emergency shock treatment
Spascupreel tablets	Cramping, colic
Traumeel tablets	Pain of all types
Vomisal drops	Vomiting
Wound Balm spray	
(Dr. Schaette)	Wound disinfection

When body temperatures fall below 100°F (38°C), the cause may be a hidden abscessation somewhere in the body.

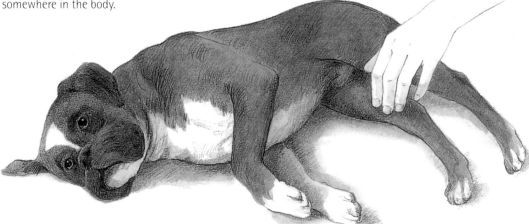

Press your fingers gently against the inside of the thigh to measure a dog's pulse.

Practical Advice

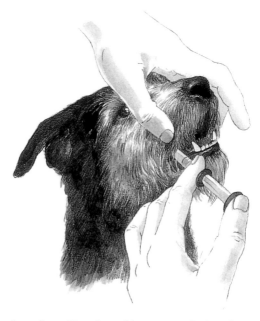

Administering Home Remedies

Even under the most favorable circumstances a dog can get sick and be in need of home remedies to get well. Many of these special medications taste or smell repulsive, and you will have to learn how to trick your patient into swallowing them. Here are some tips to help you with these tasks.

Tablets and Globules

If your dog absolutely refuses to accept pills of any sort, use a spoon to powderize them. Then, moisten your index finger, pick up the powdered medication, and wipe it off on the dog's tongue or inside the cheek. Powders dissolve very quickly, and you need not worry about them being spat right back at you.

Another method you can try is to dissolve the medication in about 2 ml of water and inject it via a plastic syringe into your dog's mouth as shown in the drawing on this page.

Drops

Administer drops by placing them directly inside the mouth with a plastic spoon. If you cannot manage this method, pull up the liquid in a small plastic syringe, and squeeze it right between the lips. If the product has a strong alcohol smell, you might dilute it with a few drops of water to reduce the distasteful smell.

Ampules

Whenever you purchase ampules with liquid medications ask your veterinarian for a prescription

Use a disposable syringe without an attached needle to administer liquid medications from ampules.

for 2 cc syringes and #2 needles. Note: Syringes must be destroyed or disposed of properly. Ask your veterinarian or pharmacist how to handle this in your area.

The manufacturer marks the ampule at the neck in order to facilitate breaking it off. Turn the indicated mark toward yourself and break the neck away from you. Place the tip of the needle at the bottom of the ampule, and pull the liquid into the syringe. Discard the needle safely, and inject the liquid directy into the dog's mouth from the plastic tip of the syringe. If you do not use the entire contents of the ampule, you can tape the top shut, and store it, standing upright, inside a little shot glass until you need to use the remainder one or two days later. These preparations do not need refrigeration.

Medications for Eyes and Ears

Nowadays you will find most eye drops in the form of small ampules containing about 1 ml of

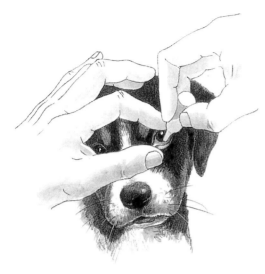

Hold the eye open with two fingers to administer eye drops.

Hold the affected ear firmly before you instill the drops.

medication. They used to be sold in 10 ml vials that expired four to six weeks after they were opened.

Hold the head of the dog up and backward, and stabilize the eye between forefinger and thumb. Then drop the medication, one drop at a time in the middle of each eye. Always treat both eyes even if only one eye is affected. Many inflammations get carried from one eye to the other. The blink reflex will automatically distribute the drops over the eye surface. When you need to administer ear medication in the form of drops, hold the outer ear with one hand while instilling the drops directy from the ampule into the ear canal. If you have not used all of the ear medication after two to three days, discard the rest.

Ointments, Tinctures, and Sprays

First, follow the instructions for the dilution of tinctures, and then apply the diluted substance for cleaning, dabbing, or irrigation of the affected skin.

Apply ointments very sparingly. Do not bandage affected areas that are treated with ointments because this causes clogging of the skin and a lack of air circulation.

When you use sprays make sure that the application yields a very thin coverage.

Practical Advice

Preventive Care

For the general health and well-being of a dog it is important to pay equal attention to aspects of husbandry as you would to body care and grooming. This includes close inspection and maintenance of the eyes, mouth, paws, and anal area.

Coat

Brushing: Your daily quota of affection can easily be combined with your grooming schedule if you do not use a scratchy brush, and you brush with loving srokes and intensity. Brushing not only removes dirt and loose hairs, it is an excellent way to stimulate healthy circulation in the skin.

Longhaired dogs must be combed before they are brushed. Remove matted hair by cutting it out.

Bathing: Unless the dog is very dirty, bathing is not necessary. Frequent bathing harms the acid balanced protective skin layer! It is important that you use a pH-neutral shampoo when you bathe your dog because this will allow thorough rinsing and removal of the detergent. The dog must be dried as thoroughly as possible, either with a towel or with a hair dryer. Allow at least two to three hours before you let the dog run outside when the weather is cool. Do not risk a cold.

Eyes

Every morning you should remove any eye secretions that might have accumulated overnight. Use a tissue and gently wipe toward the nose and down. Do not use cotton balls because lint can irritate the eyes. If the secretion is dried, do not try to pull it off, rather use a little Calendula essence to soften it first. Do not use camomile or boric acid preparations because they irritate the eyes.

Nose

Sniffing is part of a dog's natural behavior, and it gets them dirty noses. Use a wash cloth and tepid water for a simple cleanup.

Paws

It is a good idea to get into the habit of rinsing your dog's paws after every extended walk. This will help you find little stones, chewing gum, matted hair clumps, and other foreign objects. If the foot pads appear cracked, rub a small amount of Dr. Schaette ointment or plain petroleum jelly on the affected pads.

From time to time you should make sure that the hair between the pads does not grow too long. Trim it when necessary. It should not extend past the pads.

Larger, heavier dogs develop callusses because of their weight. Treat these thickened skin sections with Dr. Schaette's ointment or with petroleum jelly.

Nails

As a rule dogs keep their nails short because they walk on hard sufaces. However, there are many small breeds and old dogs who do not get enough exercise either because they are being carried or because they do not walk extensively enough. These dogs need a pedicure from time to time. Nails should not be longer than the thickness of the pads. If you attend to the nails from the beginning, you will rarely need to trim them. The use of a nail file will be sufficient. If the nails have grown too long, it is preferable if you have them taken care of by a specialist. The procedure requires great care because there are blood vessels and nerves in the tip of the nail. When you trim the nails you must be careful not to injure the blood vessels or the nerves.

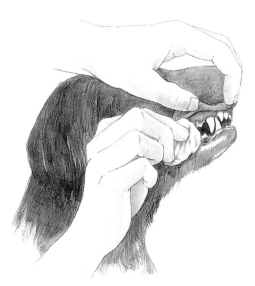

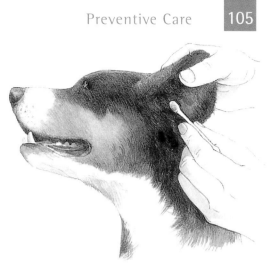

Use a wet rag with baking soda or Luvos Heilerde (mud) to clean your dog's teeth.

Use extra thick cotton swabs to clean the ears in order to protect the ear drum from injury.

Teeth

Check the teeth of your dog often and thoroughly. If you notice tartar deposits, get the teeth cleaned by a health care specialist. To prevent dental deposits you should clean them regularly with a rag on which you place a little baking soda, Luvos Heilerde (mud), or a dog toothpaste.

Giving your pet a daily dog biscuit inhibits the accumulation of deposits.

Ears

A good normal routine for the ears would consist of a weekly cleaning program. Use extra thick cotton swabs dipped in Calendula essence. If you have regular cotton swabs, wind some additional cotton around the end to make it thicker in order to protect the inner ear.

If you notice that little bunches of hair grow in the ear, you should cut them, or, if your dog lets you get away with it, pull them out carefully.

Anal and Penile Areas

You should clean the penile and anal areas after every walk. Use warm water and dry the skin well. Keep the hair in the anal area short to prevent matting and caking with fecal matter and with anal sac secretions. Also, trim the hairs growing around the tip of the penis so they are not pulled inside and cause infections (see page 61).

Practical Advice

Diets

If your dog suffers from certain metabolic disorders, you can enhance the healing process by preparing specific diets.

There are also a variety of excellent commercial diets available. Not all such foods are equally accepted by your dog though. If you choose commercial diets, try to find a variety that does not have too many chemical preservatives in it, otherwise you are just adding another burden to an already impaired organ function.

Diets for Allergies

During the first few days replace all meats with natural rice, cottage cheese or low fat cottage cheese, and vegetables. You must find out whether your dog is allergic to any of these foods. Once the symptoms recede, you can add lamb to the diet. Lamb is the lowest of all meats in protein content.

If your dog starts to itch after you add poultry or veal to the diet, discontinue those meats altogether.

If your dog tends to have allergies, you might want to discontinue dry kibbles because dry foods contain chemical preservatives that can be highly irritating to a sensitive organism. The same is true for many canned foods that contain chemicals for the purpose of color, scent, and preservation.

The healing effect of special diets is at its highest if the daily food ration is divided into 4–5 small portions that are fed throughout the day (see page 16).

Diet for Gastrointestinal Problems

Withhold food for one day and encourage the dog to drink water. During the following two days you should feed a meatless diet, preferably cooked rice, cottage cheese, and vegetables. Use chicken broth to cook the food to give it flavor.

Subsequently you can add small amounts of cooked lamb, chicken, or veal to the diet, as long as you observe improvement in the condition. Only when all symptoms are back to normal should you reintroduce the regular dog food menu.

Diet for Gastritis

Above all do not feed meats! Replace the normal diet with an emphasis on oatmeal, rice, and highly digestible grains. During the first few days allow only mucinous soups, like oatmeal or cream of wheat cooked in water. On the third day you may add meat broth or cook the soup in broth.

Once the symptoms recede, give your dog fennel, potatoes, pasta, or rice. You may add a touch of meat, but you should retain the pattern of feeding multiple small meals.

Diet for Liver Diseases

This diet should contain only small amounts of low fat meats, such as poultry, lamb, beef heart, or veal. You can add unprocessed rice, cottage cheese, and vegetables. You might want to vary this with some thick soupy cereals like oatmeal, to which you add a little fructose made from grapes.

Diet for Pancreatitis

The dog should be fed predominantly with tripe because the stomach contains nutrients that are already predigested and are, therefore, easily absorbed by your animal. In addition, you can feed your dog potatoes, rice, pasta, and low fat cottage cheese.

Diet for Kidney Disease

You should cook unprocessed rice and vegetables, and add a tiny amount of salt. To this you can add potatoes, milk diluted with water, oil of thistles, one raw egg yolk, and cottage cheese. Steamed fish fillets are also permitted. Of the meats only lamb is recommended because it contains the least protein. Make sure you are not getting mutton instead of lamb. Mutton is considerably higher in proteins. Veal may be added from time to time.

Diet for Dogs Suffering from Stone Formation

It is important to diagnose the type of stone that is being formed before you embark on a diet. A veterinarian will analyze the minerals and give you a correct diet plan.

The following table gives you a tentative guide.

Type of Stone	Avoid	Feed
Calcium	Milk, bones	Grains, meats
Oxalates	Vegetables, potatoes	Cereals, grains, fish, cooked meat
Magnesium	Uncooked meat (muscle meat)	Cooked fish and meats, rice, milk, cottage cheese

Diet for Diabetics

Increase the proportions of fresh meats, especially tripe (see pancreatitis diet), while reducing the amount of cereals and rice.

Diet for Weight Reduction

Obesity is bad for your dog's health, and it endangers the joint apparatus and the heart, especially in older dogs.

The most effective method is to cut the amount of food in half. You should avoid too much dry kibbles, and replace them with rice and vegetables. You can also cut the food to 60 percent and divide that amount into several small meals that you feed throughout the day. In addition, you need to give your dog as much exercise as possible to stimulate the metabolic activities.

practical Advice

Injuries

What dog lives without injuries? The following suggestions will help you with first aid in cases of minor injuries. If, however, your dog was involved in an accident, you need to take the animal for an office visit in order to diagnose any potential internal injuries.

Wound Dressing

Examine your dog for any skin lesions. Clip the hair carefully around the injury. A small lesion can be cleaned with diluted Calendula essence. Allow the tincture to dry, and follow with a thin coat of Dr. Schaette's Wound spray for disinfection.

All bleeding wounds must be bandaged after you have cleaned them. The best way is to place a gauze pad over the lesion, then, using a gauze bandage, wind it crosswise toward the heart.

You must make sure that the bandage is not too tight.

As first aid in all cases of injuries you need to administer Bach Flower Rescue drops (three, five, or ten drops) and, as homeopathic medication, one tablet of Arnica C30. This will prevent the animal from lapsing into a dangerous shock condition.

In all cases of pain give your animal one Traumeel tablet every fifteen minutes.

Lymphomyosot drops (three, five, or ten drops) increase the dog's own defense mechanisms. This will help the dog to fend off infections at the site of the injury.

A gaping wound must be stitched up by a veterinarian.

Bite Wounds

Any time your dog is bitten by another dog you must inspect you pet immediately for bite wounds. These bites are prone to infections from the teeth of the other dog. Absesses form quickly if the bite is not attended to (see page 76).

It would be a better idea if you had your dog looked over by a veterinarian in case the bite is so small that you did not find it.

Treat your dog immediately with Rescue drops and with one Traumeel tablet every fifteen minutes.

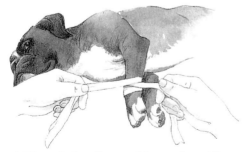

1. Wrap a 3–5 cm tie around the paw toward the heart, using a gauze bandage or something similar.

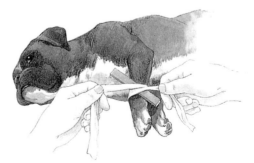

2. Place a small piece of wood or another hard object directly underneath the knot.

Profusely Bleeding Injuries

If you observe blood spouting from a wound, it is a sign that an artery was cut. In order to prevent excess loss of blood you will need to place a tourniquet bandage on the affected area. Take a clean cloth and fold it several times, then press it on the bleeding spot. While holding the cloth down tightly, bandage it in place with strips of rags or with a proper bandage. While you tie the bandage, you must keep the pressure strong enough to suppress the bleeding. Immediately take your animal to an emergency clinic!

If the bleeding is located on a paw or on the tail, you should tie off the injured vessel above the bleeding point without placing a bandage on the injury itself. (See illustrations at bottom of page 108 and this page.) If it takes a long time before you can reach the veterinarian, you need to loosen the pressure bandage for a short time every half hour.

If the bleeding is located along the belly, you need to hold a pressure compress on the bleeding spot until it stops bleeding. Then, wind a gauze bandage around the body to keep the compress in place until you reach the veterinarian.

Burns

First, cool the affected area with cold water or with ice cubes. Ice cubes are best applied by crushing them and wrapping them in a cloth or handkerchief.

For suggested medications, see page 94.

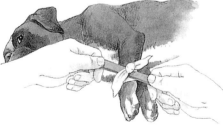

3. Turn the piece of wood just enough to stop the bleeding.

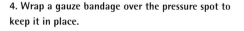

4. Wrap a gauze bandage over the pressure spot to keep it in place.

Practical Advice

Recognizing Illnesses

In many instances your dog will clearly communicate to you exactly how and where it is hurting. Never ignore these communications because they are valuable indicators for you when serious diseases might be underway.

The "Prayer" Position
It looks just like the dog is stretching, but then the dog remains down on its front legs while lifting its hind quarters as high as possible. If the dog takes this position while it is not engaged in play, there is a strong chance that the dog is suffering from pancreatic disease.

Sledding
The animal sits on its hind quarters, pulling itself forward by its front legs, and sliding the anal region along the floor.

Other dogs lick and chase their tail, and many dogs indicate difficulty in defecation. The stool may smell quite unpleasant.

In most cases the behavior points to an anal sac disorder (see page 80). However, sometimes encrusted soft stool remnants or caked up long hairs around the anus may cause the same behavior (see page 105, Anal and Penile Areas).

Extended Tail
In most dog breeds the tail hangs down beginning at the end of the vertebral column. A tail that stands up and out from the dog should arouse your immediate suspicion. The animal might also turn a circle around itself, as if trying to catch or bite its tail.

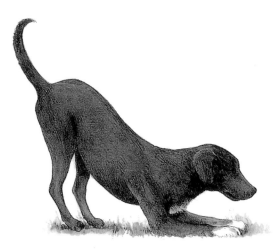

This position relieves pressure on the pancreas and is a signal of pancreatic disease.

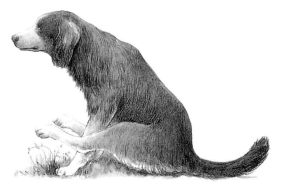

"Sledding" is most often a sign of clogged anal sacs.

This behavior is a direct indication of prostate disease (see page 69).

Head Tilt

When a dog holds its head to one side it is probably due to a foreign body lodged in the ear or by an otitis (see page 36).

Pencil Stool

The stool of the dog is of normal consistency, however, it is distinctly thin in shape, resembling a "pencil." Most commonly this typical symptom is caused by an enlargement of the prostate, by a narrowed intestinal passage due to a tumor, or by an abnormal mucosal condition of the intestinal tract.

In any case, you need to see a veterinarian.

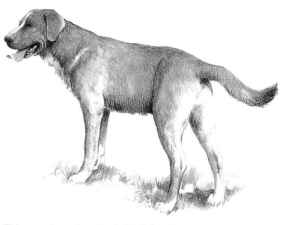

This conspicuously extended tail signals prostate disease.

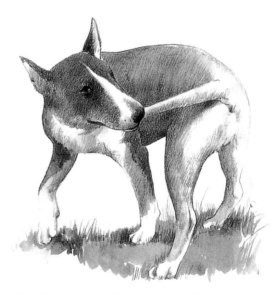

When the prostate elicits a sudden pain, the dog turns reflexively trying to bite its tail.

Home Remedies and Homeopathic Medications

This section lists all remedies and medications that are referred to in the text under the subjects of home remedies, descriptions of diseases, self-help, and preventive and convalescent care. The indications listed in the index refer specifically to the suggested applications in the text. Each formulation is, in addition, effective against a number of other symptoms. Some ingredients are designated with the *Potentiation Accord*, which indicates set homeopathic preparations in the dilutions D6, D12, D30, and D200.

Abrotanum-Injeel (Heel)
Ingredients: Homeopathic single remedy, potentiation accord
Indication: Convalescent aid, lack of appetite
Available as: Ampules, 5 pcs.

Arconitum-Injeel (Heel)
Ingredients: Homeopathic single remedy, potentiation accord
Indication: Stimulation of the body's defense mechanism, fever, infectious diseases
Available as: Ampules, 5 pcs.

Alkala (Sanum)
Ingredients: Sodium sulfate, citrate, hydrogen carb., gravel, other
Indication: For the regulation of the acid-base proportions in digestive disease
Available as: Powder, 150 g

Apis-Injeel (Heel)
Ingredients: Homeopathic single remedy, potentiation accord, 10 g
Indication: Insect stings, edema
Available as: Ampules, 5 pcs.

Apis C30 (DHU)
Ingredients: Homeopathic single remedy, in C30
Indication: Insect stings, swellings, allergies
Available as: Tablets and dilution, 20 g

Arnica C30 (DHU)
Ingredients: Homeopathic single remedy, in C30
Indication: Muscle ache, injuries, surgeries
Available as: Tablets and dilution, 70 g

Arsenicum album-Injeel (Heel)
Ingredients: Homeopathic single remedy, potentiation accord
Indication: Poisoning skin disorders, convalescent aid, diarrhea, weight loss
Available as: Ampules, 5 pcs.

ATR 9, ATR 20 (SUN)
Ingredients: Trace elements, vitamin E, electrolyte, minerals, extract of New Zealand crustaceans, other
Indication: Connective tissue fortification, ATR 9 for small dogs, ATR 20 for large dogs
Available as: Food supplement, can containing 1000 g

Basica (Protina)
Ingredients: Calcium, potassium, magnesium, copper citrate, iron, magnesiumlactate, other
Indication: For deficiencies of minerals and trace elements
Available as: Powder, 200 g

Belladonna-Injeel (Heel)
Ingredients: Homeopathic single remedy, potentiation accord
Indication: Localized inflammation, neuralgia, epilepsy
Available as: Ampules, 5 pcs.

Belladonna D12 (DHU)
Ingredients: Homeopathic single remedy, in D12
Indication: Localized inflammation
Available as: Tablets and dilution.

Berberis D12 (DHU)
Ingredients: Homeopathic single remedy, in D12
Indication: Kidney and bladder dieases
Available as: Tablets and dilution, 10 g

Biotin (Canina)
Ingredients: Vitamin H, B1, B2, B6, B12
Indication: Skin disorders, itching, hair loss
Available as: Powder, 200 g

Bryaconeel (Heel)
Ingredients: Bryonia D4, Aconitum D4, Phosphorus DS
Indication: Neuralgia, bronchitis, cough
Available as: Tablets, 50 pcs.

Bryonia-Injeel (Heel)
Ingredients: Homeopathic single remedy, potentiation accord
Indication: Pneumonia, bronchitis, inflammations
Available as: Ampules, 5 pcs.

Cactus comp. (Heel)
Ingredients: Cactus D1, Spigelia D, pot. carb. D3, Glonoinum D3, Cratagus
Indication: Age related heart problems, circulatory disorders related to heart vessels
Available as: Dilution, 30 ml

Calcium carbonicum C30 (DHU)
Ingredients: Homeopathic single remedy, in C30
Indication: Conditioning for strongly built animals, enhancement of overall condition, and bone structure
Available as: Tablets and dilution, 20 g

Calcium fluoratum C30 (DHU)
Ingredients: Homeopathic single remedy, in C30
Indication: Improvement of bones, tendons, and teeth
Available as: Tablets and Dilution, 20 g

Calcium iodatum-Injeel (Heel)
Ingredients: Homeopathic single remedy, potentiation accord
Indication: Glandular diseases
Available as: Ampules, 5 pcs.

Calendula-Essence (Weleda)
Ingredients: Marigold tincture
Indication: Wound cleansing or other cleaning
Available as: Solution, 100 ml

Cantharis D12 (DHU)
Ingredients: Homeopathic single remedy, in D2
Indication: Diseases of the kidney, bladder, urinary incontinence
Available as: Tablets and dilution, 10 g

Carbo-vegetabilis-Injeel (Heel)
Ingredients: Homeopathic single remedy, potentiation accord
Indication: Circulatory problems, dyspnea
Available as: Ampules, 5pcs.

Carminativum (Hetterich)
Ingredients: Plant extractions from chamomile, Melisse, caraway, fennel, other
Indication: Gas
Available as: Dilution, 30 ml and 100 ml

Caulophyllum C30 (DHU)
Ingredients: Homeopathic single remedy, in C30
Indication: Weak labor, uterine inertia
Available as: Tablets and dilution, 20 g

Causticum-Injeel (Heel)
Ingredients: Homeopathic single remedy, potentiation accord
Indication: Burns, weak bladder, hard warts
Available as: Ampules, 5 pcs.

Causticum comp. (Heel)
Ingredients: Caust, Sulfur, Arnica, Puls., Histamine, other
Indication: Burns
Available as: Dilution, 30 ml

Cerebrum comp. (Heel)
Ingredients: Cerebrum suis, Hyos-cyam., Gelsem., Aescul., other
Indication: Encephalitis, epilepsy, brain contusion
Available as: Ampules, 5pcs.

Chelidonium-Injeel (Heel)
Ingredients: Homeopathic single remedy, potentiation accord
Indication: Liver-gall bladder disease
Available as: Ampules, 5pcs.

China-Injeel (Heel)
Ingredients: Homeopathic single remedy, potentiation accord
Indication: Convalescent aid, reduces weakness
Available as: Ampules, 5 pcs.

Colocynthis-Hcc. (Heel)
Ingredients: Colocynthis, Graphalium polyceph
Indication: Neuralgia, problems in the pelvic bone structures
Available as: Dilution, 30 ml

Comius Hcc. (Heel)
Ingredients: Cocculus, petroleum
Indication: Car sickness
Available as: Dilution, 30 ml

Conium-Injeel (Heel)
Ingredients: Homeopathic single
remedy, potentiation accord
Indication: Testicular indurations,
gerontological aid
Available as: Ampules, 5 pcs.

Conjunctisan A (VitOrgan)
Ingredients: Macromolecular
organ substances (cytoplasm
therapy)
Indication: Degenerative eye
disorders
Available as: Vials, 20 pcs.

Cor comp. (Heel)
Ingredients: Crataegus, Arnica,
Cactus, Glonoinum, other
Indication: Heart diseases
Available as: Ampules, 5 pcs.

**Cosmochema Cough Drops
(Cosmochema)**
Ingredients: Ipetacuanha, Tartarus
stib, Spongla, Phosphorus, other
Indication: Colds and flulike condi-
tions with cough and bronchitis
Available as: Dilution, 30 ml and
100 ml

**Cosmochema Gastrointestinal
Drops (Cosmochema)**
Ingredients: Pulsatilla, Belladonna,
Nux vom., Colocynthis, Carbo-
veg., other
Indication: Gastritis, heartburn
Available as: Dilution, 30 ml and
100 ml

**Cosmochema Liver-Gall
Bladder Drops (Cosmochema)**
Ingredients: Chelidon, Lycopod,
Carduus mar., Nux vom,
Mandragora, Momordica,
Veratrum, other
Indication: Stimulating liver and
biliary functions
Available as: Dilution, 30 ml and
100 ml

**Cosmochema Skin Function
Drops (Cosmochema)**
Ingredients: Graphites, Sulfur,
Histamine, Thuja, Thallium, other
Indication: Skin function
disorders, eczema, hair loss
Available as: Dilution, 30 ml and
100 ml

Cralonin (Heel)
Ingredients: Crataegus, Spigelia,
potassium carbon.
Indication: Age related heart
problems, myocardial damage,
Available as: Dilution, 30 ml

**Crataegus-Plantaplex
(Steigerwald)**
Ingredients: Crataegus, Arnica,
CactusSolidago, other
Indication: Age related heart
problems, congestive heart failure
with edema
Available as: Dilution, 50 ml

Croton D12 (DHU)
Ingredients: Homeopathic single
remedy, D12
Indication: Itching, scrotal
eczema, neuralgia
Available as: Tablets and dilution,
10 ml

Dental-Can (Canina)
Ingredients: Chlorhexidin,
Ethyl-alcohol
Indication: Mouth odors,
gingivitis
Available as: Solution, 250 ml

Dermisal (WeraVet)
Ingredients: Sulfur C30
Indication: General detoxification,
skin function disorders
Available as: Dilution, 20 ml

Diarrheel (Heel)
Ingredients: Argent. nitr.,
Podophyl., Veratrum, Arsen alb.,
other
Indication: Diarrhea
Available as: Tablets, 50 pcs.

Discus comp. (Heel)
Ingredients: Discus intervert.
suis, Cartilago suis, Cimicifuga,
Ledum, Colocynthis Aesculus,
other
Indication: Dachshund paralysis,
disc prolapse
Available as: Ampules, 5 pcs.

**Dr. Schaette Wandsalbe
(wound balm) (Schaette)**
Ingredients: Cetiol, Phenol
Indication: Scabby encrusted
wounds, dry eczema
Available as: Ointment, 75 g
(see a veterinarian for this)

**Dr. Schaette Wandbalsam-
Spray (wound spray)
(Schaette)**
Ingredients: Perubalsam, Thyme
oil, Camomile, Ringeiblume, oak
bark, other

Indication: Disinfection of wounds
Available as: Spray, 100 ml
(see a veterinarian for this)

Dulcamara C30 (DHU)
Ingredients: Homeopathic single
remedy, in C30
Indication: Wet weather
conditions, rheumatism, soft
warts
Available as: Tablets and dilution,
20 g

Dulcamara-Injeel (Heel)
Ingredients: Homeopathic single
remedy, potentiation accord
Indication: Wet weather
conditions, soft warts
Available as: Ampules, 5 pcs.

Dysenteral (WeraVet)
Ingredients: Arsen alb., Rheum,
Podophyllum, in C30
Indication: Diarrhea
Available as: Dilution, 20 ml

Echinacea comp. (Heel)
Ingredients: Echinac., Aconit.,
Lachesis, Bryon, Grippe-Nosode,
pyrogen, Gelsem, Euphorbium,
other
Indication: Stimulation of the
body's defense mechanism
Available as: Ampules, 5 pcs.

Engystol (Heel)
Ingredients: Vincetoxicum, Sulfur
Indication: Detoxification,
stimulation of the body's own
defenses
Available as: Ampules, 5 pcs.

Euphorbium comp. (Heel)
Ingredients: Euphorb., Pulsat.,
Luffa, Mucocsa nasalis suis, other
Indication: Colds, sinus conditions
Available as: Ampules, 5 pcs.

Euphrasia-Eye Drops (Wala)
Ingredients: Euphrasia D2, Rosae
aetherol D7
Indication: Conjunctivitis
Available as: Vials, 5 pcs.

Febrisal (WeraVet)
Ingredients: Aconit, Echinacea,
Lache-sis, in C30
Indication: Fever, strengthen
body's own defense mechanism
Available as: Dilution, 20 ml

Flor de Piedra D12 (DHU)
Ingredients: Homeopathic single
remedy, in D12
Indication: Liver bile diseases,
parasitism, Hamamelis
Available as: Tablets and dilution,
10 g

Formel-Z (Biopet)
Formula-Z
Ingredients: Yeast, vitamin B1,
other
Indication: Natural tick prevention
Available as: Tablets, 125 g
(see a veterinarian for this)

Frubiase-Calcium (Boehringer)
Ingredients: Calcium carbonate,
citric acid
Indication: Cacium deficiency
problems, allergies, disposition to
cramps
Available as: Ampules, 20 pcs.

Gastricumeel (Heel)
Ingredients: Pulsat., Nux vom.,
Carbo-veg., Arg. nitr., other
Indication: Stomach ulcers,
heartburn
Available as: Tablets, 50 pcs.

Gelsemium-Hec (Heel)
Ingredients: Gelsemium,
Cimicifusa, Rhus tox.
Indication: Problems of the neck
bones
Available as: Dilution, 30 ml

Gerontamin (Pierre Fabre)
Ingredients: Gelatine, L-Cystin,
Retinolacetat, vitamin A
Indication: Arthrosis
Available as: Bags, 28 pcs.

Graphites-Injeel (Heel)
Ingredients: Homeopathic single
remedy, potentiation accord
Indication: Dry skin eczema,
obesity
Available as: Ampules, 5 pcs.

Gripp Heel (Heel)
Ingredients: Aconit., Bryonia,
Laches, Eupator, Phosphorus
Indication: Flulike infections
Available as: Tablets, 50 pcs.

Hamamelis Salbe (ointment) (Heel)
Ingredients: Hamameis extract
Indication: Skin irritations, dry
skin, anal sac inflammation
Available as: Ointment, 20 g

Hamamelis Tincture (Weleda)
Ingredients: Hamamelis
Indication: Wound dressing
Available as: Tincture, 100 ml

Heelax (Heel)
Ingredients: Aloe, Rheum,
Frangula
Indication: Constipation
Available as: Dragees, 30 pcs.

Hepar comp. (Heel)
Ingredients: Hepar suis, China,
Lycopod., Chelidon, Carduus,
Sulfur, Fel tauri, other
Indication: Liver disease, skin
disorders
Available as: Ampules, 5 pcs.

Hepar sulfuris-Injeel (Heel)
Ingredients: Homeopathic single
remedy, potentiation accord
Indication: Purulent conditions,
panaritium (see page 121)
Available as: Ampules, 5 pcs.

Hepeel (Heel)
Ingredients: Lycopod., Chelidon.,
China, Carduus, Veratr., other
Indication: Liver function
disorders
Available as: Tablets, 50 pcs.

Hormeel (Heel)
Ingredients: Senecio, Puls, Sepia,
Ignat., Cyclamen, other
Indication: Disorders of the female
hormone system
Available as: Dilution, 30 ml

Husteel (Heel)
Ingredients: Arsen. jod, Bellad
Caust Scilla, Cuprum ac.

Indication: Cough, Bronchitis
Available as: Dilution, 30 ml

Hydrastis-Injeel (Heel)
Ingredients: Homeopathic single
remedy, potentiation accord
Indication: Mucosal disorders,
stringy mucus
Aavailable as: Ampules, 5 pcs.

Hypericum-Injeel (Heel)
Ingredients: Homeopathic single
remedy, potentiation accord
Indication: Neuralgia, nerve pain
Available as: Ampules, 5 pcs.

Hypericum D4 (DHU)
Ingredients: Homeopathic single
remedy, in D4
Indication: Neurologic diseases,
burns
Available as: Tablets and dilution,
10 g

Ichtholan 20% (Ichthyol)
Ingredients: Ammonium
bitumino-sulfonat
Indication: Inflammatory skin
conditions, abscesses
Available as: Ointment, 40 g

Ignatia-Injeel (Heel)
Ingredients: Homeopathic single
remedy, potentiation accord
Indication: Nervousness,
psychological weaknesses
Available as: Ampules, 5 pcs.

Keratisal (WeraVet)
Ingredients: Belladonna,
Euphrasia, in C30
Indication: Conjunctivitis
Available as: Dilution, 20 ml

Kryosotum-Injeel (Heel)
Ingredients: Homeopathic single
remedy, potentiation accord
Indication: Mucosal inflammations,
malodorous discharges
Available as: Ampules, 5 pcs.

Lachesis-Injeel (Heel)
Ingredients: Homeopathic single
remedy, potentiation accord
Indication: Infections, left remedy
(see page 121)
Available as: Ampules, 5 pcs.

Ladlesis D30 (DHU)
Ingredients: Homeopathic single
remedy, in D30
Indication: Bleeding, ulcers,
suppurative conditions
Available as: Tablets and dilution,
10 g

**Luvos Heilerde Innerlich
(Heilerde Ges. Luvos Just)**
Ingredients: Gravel, Calc., Alum.,
Magnes, Pot. oxide, other
Indication: Gastrointestinal
disorders, teeth cleaning
Available as: Powder, 220 g

Lycoaktin (Steigerwald)
Ingredients: Crataegus, Leonuri
card., Lycopi Extracts, other
Indication: Hyperthyroidism
Available as: Tablets, 50 pcs.

Lycopodium-Injeel (Heel)
Ingredients: Homeopathic single
remedy, potentiation accord
Indication: Liver and gall bladder
disorders, right remedy,
(see page 122)
Available as: Ampules, 5 pcs.

Lymphomyosot (Heel)
Ingredients: Ferrum jos., Aranea diad., Juglans Veronica, other
Indication: Lymphatic disorders, glandular dysfunctions and enlargements
Available as: Dilution, 30 ml.

Magnesium-Verla (Verla)
Ingredients: Magn.-hydrogen-glutamat, Magn.-citrat, other
Indication: Tetany, pancreatitis, cirrhosis of the liver
Available as: Dragees, 20 pcs.

Melaleuka (Krieger-GmbH)
Ingredients: Melaleuca oil (tea tree)
Indication: gingivitis
Available as: Oil containing liquid, 10 ml (see a veterinarian for this)

Mercurius-Injeel (Heel)
Ingredients: Homeopathic single remedy, potentiation accord
Indication: Gingivitis
Available as: Ampules, 5 pcs.

Mucosa comp. (Heel)
Ingredients: Arg. nitr., Bellad., Phosph., Puls, other
Indication: Mucosal disorders
Available as: Ampules, 5 pcs.

Myristica sebifera D12 (DHU)
Ingredients: Homeopathic single remedy, in D12
Indication: Abscess formation
Available as: Tablets and dilution, 10 g

Natrium (sodium) muriaticum-Injeel (Heel)
Ingredients: Homeopathic single remedy, potentiation accord
Indication: Emaciation despite food intake, canned food diet
Available as: Ampules, 5 pcs.

Nervoheel (Heel)
Ingredients: Ignatia, Sepia, Psorin., Kal brom Zincum, other
Indication: Psychological imbalance, neuroses
Available as: Tablets, 50 pcs.

Nettisabal (Iso)
Ingredients: Populus, Hyosyamus, Puls., Sabal ser., other
Indication: Prostate enlargement, cystitis
Available as: Dilution, 50 ml

Nux vomica-Hcc (Heel)
Ingredients: Nux vom., Bryonia, Lycopod, Colocynthis
Indication: Stomach, intestine, liver disorders, gas
Available as: Dilution, 30 ml

Nux-vomica D6 (DHU)
Ingredients: Homeopathic single remedy, in D6
Indication: Dachshund paralysis syndrome, constipation, poisoning
Available as: Tablets and dilution, 10 g

Okoubaka D4 (DHU)
Ingredients: Homeopathic single remedy, in D4
Indication: Accumulation of toxins, poisoning

Available as: Tablets and dilution,10 g

Paeonia (Heel)
Ingredients: Paeonia, Graphit., Sulfur, Hamamelis, other
Indication: Anal sac inflammation, hemorrhoids
Available as: Tablets, 50 pcs.

Perenterol (Thiemann)
Ingredients: Saccharomyces cerev., lactose, Saccharose
Indication: Diarrhea
Available as: Capsules, 20 pcs.

Phytolacca-Injeel (Heel)
Ingredients: Homeopathic single remedy, potentiation accord
Indication: Mastitis, tonsillitis
Available as: Ampules, 5 pcs.

PichiPichi C30 (DHU)
Ingredients: Homeopathic single remedy, in C30
Indication: Calcification of the vertebral column (together with Dulcamara and Rhus tox)
Available as: Dilution, 20 g

Platinum C200 (DHU)
Ingredients: Homeopathic single remedy, in C200
Indication: Increased sexual drive
Available as: Dilution, 20 g

Pro-Aller (Pekana)
Ingredients: Comoclad Ailanthus, Euphras, Okoubaka, other
Indication: Allergic reactions, detoxification (internal purification)
Available as: Dilution, 20 ml

Prostagutt (Schwabe)
Ingredients: Sabal serr., Populi trem, Urticae, other
Indication: Prostate enlargement
Available as: Dilution, 50 ml

Psorinoheel (Heel)
Ingredients: Psorin., Medorrhin., Sulfur, Thuja, Luesin, other
Indication: Skin and liver disorders, internal unspecific purification
Available as: Dilution, 30 ml

Pulsatilla-Injeel (Heel)
Ingredients: Homeopathic single remedy, potentiation accord
Indication: Disorders of the female hormonal system, pseudopregnancy
Available as: Ampules, 5 pcs.

Pyrogenium-Injeel (Heel)
Ingredients: Homeopathic single remedy, potentiation accord
Indication: Recurring skin disorders, purulent conditions, fever
Available as: Ampules, 5 pcs.

Reneel (Heel)
Ingredients: Berberis, Canthar., Sabal serr., Caust., other
Indication: Kidney and bladder disorders, stone formation
Available as: Tablets, 50 pcs.

Rescue-Cream (Bach Flowers)
Ingredients: Clemat., Impa., Helianthemum-Numm., other
Indication: Burns, injuries
Available as: Cream, 27 g

Rhus-toxicodendron C30 (DHU)
Ingredients: Homeopathic single remedy, in C30
Indication: Joint problems that are aggravated during cold and wet conditions
Available as: Tablets and Dilution, 20 g

Rumisal (WeraVet)
Ingredients: Nux vomica, C30
Indication: Digestive disorders, Dachshund paralysis
Available as: Dilution, 20 g

Secale-cornutum C30 (DHU)
Ingredients: Homeopathic single remedy in C30
Indication: Uterine inertia (weak labor)
Available as: Tablets and dilution, 20 g

Sepia-Injeel (Heel)
Ingredients: Homeopathic single remedy, single potentiation
Indication: Disorders of female hormone balance
Available as: Ampules, 5 pcs.

Silicea-Injeel (Heel)
Ingredients: Homeopathic single remedy, single potentiation
Indication: Connective tissue impairment, skin disorders
Available as: Ampules, 5 pcs.

Solidago comp. (Heel)
Ingredients: Solidago, Berb., Peyelon suis., Cantharis, other
Indication: Diseases of the kidneys and urinary tract
Available as: Ampules, 5 pc.

Spascupreel (Heel)
Ingredients: Coloeynthis, Chamom., Cuprum, Gelsem., Magn. phosphor., Veratrum, other
Indication: Cramps of all types
Available as: Tablets, 50 pcs.

Spongia-Injeel (Heel)
Ingredients: Homeopathic single remedy, single potentiation
Indication: Cough, thyroid disorders, heart problems
Available as: Ampules, 5 pcs.

Staphisagria-Injeel (Heel)
Ingredients: Homeopathic single remedy, potentiation accord
Indication: Irritability, sties, cut injuries
Available as: Ampules, 5 pcs

Staphylosal (WeraVet)
Ingredients: Hepar sulfuris, C30
Indication: Purulent conditions, abscess formation
Available as: Dilution, 20 ml

Sulfur-Injeel (Heel)
Ingredients: Homeopathic single remedy, single potentiation
Indication: Itching, skin disorders
Available as: Ampules, 5 pcs.

Sulfur C30 (DHU)
Ingredients: Homeopathic single remedy, in C30
Indication: Itching, skin disorders
Available as: Tablets and dilution, 20 g

Syzygium comp. (Heel)
Ingredients: Syzygium, Secale corn, Lycopod, sod. sulf., other
Indication: Adult-onset diabetes
Available as: Dilution, 30 ml

Tanacet-Heel (Hcc)
Ingredients: Tanacelum, Artemis vulg., Serpyllum, other
Indication: Deworming
Available as: Dilution, 30 ml

Tartephedreel (Heel)
Ingredients: Tartar. stib., Bellad., Sod. sulf. Arsen. jod., other
Indication: Bronchitis, cough
Available as: Dilution, 30 ml

Thuja-Injeel (Heel)
Ingredients: Homeopathic single remedy, potentiation accord
Indication: Cauliflower warts, skin diseases
Available as: Ampules, 5 pcs.

Thuja D30 (DHU)
Ingredients: Homeopathic single remedy, in D30
Indication: Cauliflower warts, poisoning
Available as: Tablets and dilution, 10 g

Thyreoidea comp. (Heel)
Ingredients: Galium, Conium, calc. fluorat, Thyreoidea suis, Spongia, other
Indication: Malfunction of the thyroid gland
Available as: Ampules, 5 pcs.

Toxex (Pelcana)
Ingredients: Apis, Hydrastis Okoubaka, Galium, Vlcetox, other
Indication: Unspecific detoxification
Available as: Dilution, 20 ml

Traumeel (Heel)
Ingredients: Arnica, Calend., Hamamel., Bellad., Hepar sulf., Hypcricum, other
Indication: Injuries and pain of all types
Available as: Dilution, 30 ml; tablets, 50 pcs.; ointment, 50 g; ampules, 5 pcs.

Urtica-urens D6, C30 (DHU)
Ingredients: Homeopathic single remedy, in D6 or C30
Indication: Excess lactation: D6, lack of lactation: C30
Available as: D6 tablets and dilution, 10 g; C30 tablets and dilution, 20 g

Veratrum-Hcc (Heel)
Ingredients: Veratrum, Aloe, Rheum, Tormentilla
Indication: Cardiovasc. failure
Available as: Dilution, 30 ml

Vertigoheel (Heel)
Ingredients: Cocculus, Conium, Ambra, Petroleum
Indication: Dizziness
Available as: Tablets, 50 pcs.

Vomisal (WeraVet)
Ingredients: Ipecacuanha, C30
Indication: Vomiting
Available as: Dilution, 20 ml

Zeel (Heel)
Ingredients: Cartilago suis D2, Funiculus umbilicalis D2, Rhus tox, Arnica, Symphyt., other
Indication: Arthritis, arthrosis and other joint problems
Available as: Tablets, 50 pcs.; ampules, 5 pcs.

Bach Flowers

There are 38 individual flower essences as well as the so-called "Rescue drops." The flower extracts are available, without prescription, in 10 ml vials in health food stores and homeopathic pharmacies. Rescue drops also come in 20 ml vials. In addition, there are a number of flower mixtures available. The essences may be based in water or in alcohol.

The individual flowers are as follows: Agrimony, Aspen, Beech, Centaury, Ceranto, Cherry Plum, Chestnut Bud, Chicory, Clematis, Crab Apple, Elm, Gentian, Gorse, Heather, Holly, Honeysuckle, Hornbeam, Impatiens, Larch, Mimulus, Mustard, Oak, Olive, Pine, Red Chestnut, Vervain, Vine, Walnut, Water Violet, White Chestnut, Wild Oat, Wild Rose, Willow.

Glossary

Acute Processes
Sudden, quick, severe onset

Adenoma
Benign tumor originating in glandular tissue

Affected
diseased

Allergy
Hypersensitive reaction of the body to certain substances

Anaphylaxis
Severe generalized allergic reaction to medication

Apathy
Lack of response to external stimuli

Aphta
Thrush

Bioresonance analysis
Laboratory analysis based on measuring the body's physio-logical energy field. It implies that disorders are recognizable before they become manifest as diseases. Diagnostic procedures are performed on tufts of hair or on a drop of blood. This analysis also enables a determination of specific medications that are needed to return the body to its normal, heathful amplitude.

Callus
Thickening of new bone tissue in a fracture line

Chondrodystrophy
Inherited defect of cartilage formation

Color therapy
Healing processes that are induced by exposing the patient to colored lights

Combination remedy
Homeopathic medication that consists of several homeopathic single remedies

Conditioning therapy
Stabilization or regulation of the general condition of a living being

Congestive heart failure
Lack of breath due to increased lung pressure because of circulatoy insufficiency

Conjunctivitis
Inflammation of the mucous membrane that lines the eyelids and is reflected onto the eyeball

Convalescing medication
Treatment to enhance recovery

Cytoplasm therapy
An elegant version of fresh-cell therapy. The cytoplasm is extracted exclusively. This cellular substance boosts the regenerative functions of the organism. In this extraction process foreign proteins are

removed because they are frequently the causes of allergies in other cell therapies.

Degeneretion
Deterioration of an organ or substance

Desensitization
Injection of a dog's own blood in order to treat unresolved allergies. Used in cases where multiple allergies exist.

Diabetic coma
State of unconsciousness due to excessive blood sugar levels

Dilution
Medicinal substance in liquid form

Disposition
Genetic susceptibility to diseases

Ectoparasite
Parasite living on the external surface (usually skin, hair) of the dog

Edema
Fluid accumulation in tissues

Encephalitis
Inflammation of the brain

Endoparasite
Parasites living in internal organ tissues of the dog
(see Parasite)

Energy field of the body

The frequency that surrounds a body, which is used in bioresonance analysis to find wavelengths that deviate from the norm, and which are considered potential disease-causing changes, that are measurable before they manifest as organic illnesses

Euthanasia

Humane killing by injection of anesthetic drugs

Hip dysplasia

Hereditary deformation of the hip joint

Homeopathic acute primary reaction

Initial intense reaction to a homeopathic medication

Homeopathic high potency

Homeopathic remedy diluted above D30 (see Potentized)

Homeopathic potentized cell preparation

A cellular substance that was diluted (potentiated) by homeopathic standards

Homeopathic single remedy

Homeopathic medicine formulated from one single substance and set at one specific potency

Infusion therapy

Fluid injection by a slow drip method

Initiation of healing

Use of a natural product for the purpose of stimulating the body's own healing response

Irritating discharge

A discharge that creates sores upon contact with the skin or other surfaces

Left remedies

Medications that are formulated specifically for the organs on the left side of the body

Lung edema

Accumulation of serous fluids in the lung tissue

Lymph

Alkaline fluid in the lymphatic vessels. Colorless, clear, except in intestinal areas where fats contribute to a milky color.

Materially manifest

A disease has established itself in the material organism, the body

Meridian

Chinese medical term referring to the yin and yang pathways. Considered streams of energy and lines of acupuncture points.

Mild discharge

Secretions that do not irritate the skin

Neutering (Spaying, Castration)

Surgical removal of male or female reproductive organs

(male: testis; female: ovaries, uterus)

Nosode therapy

A natural treatment procedure that operates under the principle of "like" cures "like." Substances derived from a diseased organism are administered into a patient suffering from a like disease. This serves to eliminate the disease entity from the body.

Orthopedic disorders

Disorders involving locomotive structures of the body, especially the skeleton, muscles, joints, and tendons

Panaris

Inflammation of the skin fold around the nail

Parasite

An organism that lives within, upon, or at the expense of another organism

Pathogen

A microorganism capable of producing disease

Peripheral

Outside, at the margin

Pleurisy

Inflammation of the serous membrane that enfolds the lungs

Polyarthritis

Inflammation of several joints simultaneously

Potentized formulation
Natural remedy that was prepared
by homeopathic procedures, i.e.,
diluted (potentized)

Recidivism
Recurrence of a previously
contracted disease

Resistance to therapy
The organism does not respond to
therapeutic measures

Right remedies
Medications that are specifically
formulated for the organs of the
right side of the body

Secondary infection
Infection, superimposed over a
primary one where the first
infection caused the susceptibility
for the secondary infection

Sepsis
Generalized bacterial infection

Sputum
Substance expelled by coughing
or clearing the throat

Sterilization
Severance of the vas deferens
(male), and of the oviduct
(female)

Suppurative
Producing or associated with
the generation of pus

Symptoms
Any perceptible change in the
body or its function that indicates
disease

Syndrome
A group of symptoms typical for
a disease

Tetany
Spasms that are associated with
a tetanus bacillus infection

Thrush
White patches of ulcers or
inflammation in the mouth or
throat

Toxin
A poisonous substance of animal
or plant origin. Toxins affect the
metabolism by overburdening the
detoxification pathways.

Vial
Small plastic ampule, which
contains a small amount (usually
1 ml) of medicine (e.g., eye drops)

Warts
Benign skin growths that are
usually caused by a virus

Index

Useful Literature

Brennan, Mary L., DVM, *The New Natural Dog.*
   Penguin, New York.
Brennan, Mary L., DVM, and Norma Eckroate, *The
   Natural Dog: A Complete Guide for Caring Owners,*
   NAL/Dutton, New York, 1994.
de Bairacli-Levy, Juliette, *The Complete Herbal
   Handbook for the Dog and Cat.* Arco Publishing, New
   York, 1991.
Harper, Joan, *The Healthy Cat and Dog Cookbook.* E.P.
   Dutton, New York.
Pitcairn, Richard H., DVM, and Susan Hubble Pitcairn,
   *Natural Health
   Care for Dogs and Cats.*
   Rodale Press, Emmaus, PA.
Stein, Diane, *Natural Healing for Dogs and Cats.*
   Crossing Press, Freedom, CA, 1993.
Vithoulkas, George, *The Science of Homeopathy.*
   Random House, Inc., New York, 1980.

Useful Addresses

● American Holistic Veterinarian Medical Association
2214 Old Emmorton Road
Bel Air, MD 21015
(410) 569-0795 (nationwide referrals)

● International Veterinarian Acupuncture Society
c/o Meredith Snader, DVM
Executive Director
RD #4, Box 216
Chester Springs, PA 19425
(215) 827-7245

● International Foundation for Homeopathy
2366 Eastlake Avenue E.
Suite 301
Seattle, WA 98102
(206) 324-8230

● National Center for Homeopathy
801 North Fairfax Street, Suite 306
Alexandria, VA 22314
(703) 548-7790

● Nelson Bach, USA, Ltd.
Wilmington Technology Park
100 Research Drive
Wilmington, MA 01887-4406
(800) 334-0843

The Author

Petra Stein grew up with dogs and cats. She received her training and her diplomate as "Holistic Animal Health Care Provider" in Gesenkirchen, Germany, at the German Association for Holistic Health Care Providers. She is a member of this association. Since 1986 she has had a dog and cat practice in Munich, Germany. She has taught at several vocational schools in and around Munich. She is also the author of several books on the subject of natural health care for dogs.

Publication Data

Published originally under the title *Naturheilpraxis HUNDE*
©1996 by Gräfe und Unzer Verlag GmbH, München
English translation ©Copyright 1997 by Barron's Educational Series, Inc.

All inquiries should be addressed to:
Barron's Educational Series, Inc.
250 Wireless Boulevard
Hauppauge, NY 11788

International Standard Book No. 0-7641-0122-6

Library of Congress Catalog Card No. 97-13990

Library of Congress Cataloging-in-Publication Data
Stein, Petra.
    [Naturheil Praxis Hunde. English]
    Natural health care for your dog / Petra Stein.
       p. cm.
    Includes bibliographical references (p. 127) and indexes.
    ISBN 0-7641-0122-6
      1. Dogs. 2. Dogs—Health. 3. Dogs—Diseases—Alternative treatment. I. Title.
    SF427.S8313   1997
    636.7'089—dc21   97-13990
                                                  CIP

Printed in Hong Kong.

9 8 7 6 5 4 3 2 1